GREAT BODY WHILE TRAVELING

An easy step-by-step guide to getting into great shape while traveling to exotic countries

HONESTY: free of deceit and untruthfulness; sincere
"He spoke with convincing honesty towards her"

Chris R. Rea

ReaShape

ISBN: 978-0-615-40865-1
reashape.com

The nutritional and health information in this book is based on the author's experiences. It is intended only as a guide and it not meant to replace the advice of a physician, dietician, physical therapist or other health professional. Always seek competent professional help if you have concerns about the appropriateness of this information for you.

Printed in the United States of America.

Acknowledgements

My family in the U.S and my extended family in Spain are the people who opened up a whole world of travel and culture to me. They made tremendous sacrifices to make that dream come true.

– Chris Rea

Contents

Chapter 1: Fun, Priority #1   7

Chapter 2: Business Before Pleasure   9

Chapter 3: Different Workouts for Different Places   13

Chapter 4: Eating and Training Abroad   31

    Spain

    Portugal

    Italy

    Greece

    Albania

    Montenegro

    Bosnia

    Croatia

Disclaimer

Exercise at your own risk.

Please practice extreme caution and care when finding a place or item to perform your fitness routines when not in a gym. Make sure that whatever it is that you are holding on, leaning on, or resting against is solid and can support your weight or pressure applied to.

Chapter 1: Fun, Priority #1

Hello everyone just let me start off this book by saying thank you so much for being one of my valued readers. This means a lot to me. Writing this book was of huge interest to me because looking fit and having a great time I feel should go hand in hand. Unfortunately most fitness gurus and experts have a different philosophy towards health and fitness. However if it works for you then that method is great! Never would I claim to be better than everyone else in this field, not at all. Actually on the contrary. Granted, I absolutely love what I do and really enjoy learning more and more. It seems that the more I learn the more I realize that I could learn so much more! Have I had success as a competitive athlete, personal trainer, coach, and nutritionist? Of course I have but I could always improve to the next level and knowing that gives me the drive to want to continue learning without ever stopping. When it comes to learning and improving, "sky is the limit!"

Many experts become complacent once they experience success. What happens later on is that much of what they have learned becomes out dated. Even worse off is even though their methods are outdated they continue using them the same way without ever wanting to reinvent or upgrade their talents to modern times because of either pride or complacency.

However in my case this does not apply because I constantly remain humble, am eager to accept constructive criticism and stay driven to learn more and better myself in everyway possible. Improvement and fun equal quality of life. This is why I am writing this book today to show everyone that it is possible, to succeed and have fun at the same time. More specifically what I mean is that you can create a great body while partying and enjoying life at the same time! Trust me, I am living proof of this because fitness and fun was the core of my life (often a little too much that sometimes causing me trouble). As a child my Dad labeled me "Good time Charlie" to him this was not at all a compliment but rather expressing his frustration towards my "different" priorities in life or the way I was living. For me some way and some how I managed to eat right and exercise regardless of where I was, whether being a party, a vacation at a country half round the world, , as a competitive athlete, whatever, having a great time and being in great shape was something I needed to maintain always, everywhere. To me being in shape was great and being able to take that body to another beach in the Mediterranean, party, or vacation was even better because in any of those places you will have a better time if your happy with your body, you will carry yourself with more of a "swagger" and be more confident hence you will enjoy more! Everyone believes that in order to build a great body many quality of life decreasing sacrifices need to be made, this is only partially true. Yes, many sacrifices are required but quality of life doesn't need to decrease at all.

To me it makes no sense whatsoever to have a great body, be so proud of it but not be able to completely enjoy it and even show it off a bit. Let's be honest here because all of us both women and men want to constantly do 1 thing always, and that's "turn heads" meaning attract the opposite sex. Most people try to attract the opposite sex by dressing well, wearing perfumes or colognes, raise their financial status, wearing jewelry, driving flashy cars, and even receiving the red carpet treatment everywhere such as restaurants, lounges, airports, etc. Oh, and by the way, having a fit body will actually help you achieve that red carpet status because being in shape gives you more positive energy and open minded attitude to help you want to achieve goals, all types of positive goals! Also when you're in shape and you carry yourself with the perfect combination of confidence and humility. This is definitely a goal because this combination is much more acceptable and appreciated by the general public. Let's face it, nobody appreciates a braggart. People don't appreciate a person who flashes their money or uses their muscle or looks to manipulate and or get their way. Now when a man with a muscular body or a woman with stunning looks acts as if they never had the looks or muscular body now that comes across as impressive to where even more doors will open for these people! People appreciate humility and they even try to go that extra mile to assist that humble person, especially when they have so many temptations not to be humble! They always say that the only way to really know somebody's personality is give them success and power and then see how they act because only very few will remain humble and be the same person they were before they had the power. Excuse me for drifting away from the main purpose of this book but believe it or not the psychology I have been explaining to you is to help you understand the mechanics and foundation which will help you maintain and or build a great body. The psychology will further fuel your desire and motivation.

Ok, so let's go, have fun, live it up, party, and build a great body too! It's all possible! I am about to show you the way!

Chapter 2: Business Before Pleasure

Before we can even think about being a "Good Time Charlie" we must first have a reason to celebrate meaning let's first get into shape! What good is the dessert without eating the main course, right? Of course we would all love to have a good time always but before this can happen, work needs to be done. By laying the necessary ground work first by getting into shape and then the rest is simple! What I mean is that the fruits of your work are way more appreciated. Think of dieting all week and waiting for that cheat meal on Sunday! That steak or cheesecake or whatever else you couldn't eat during the week is way more enjoyable! It's good to discipline yourself with your diet because not only does that cheat food taste so much better because you can only eat it sparingly but by disciplining yourself with your diet you see progress in your physique and you also increase your confidence in achieving goals. That ability, that test of fortitude, grit, that willingness to suffer is so valuable you could never begin to imagine. Aside from helping you create a nice physique it can help you accomplish so much more! Having that grade "A" physique opens the doors to so much more in life! You will see for yourself and soon be agreeing with me.

Dedication, desire and determination, the three D's are the primary ingredients you will need for us to get started. "Taking care of business" translates into "sweat" and get used to sweating because the results you're looking for in your body's appearance will soon follow. Resistance exercise is necessary however I have so many workout routines made to facilitate your preference and lifestyle. Depending on your schedule and how often you will train a workout routine is available. I have devised workouts that exercise your entire body in either a day or in seven days.

Ok if you can only train once a week that's fine because I have a workout routine that will exercise your entire body that day. If you can only train twice in a week I have a great full body exercise routine for that also, training your lower body one day and your upper body the other day. If you can only exercise three days per week, or four, five, six and seven days per week that's quite alright because I have a full body workout routine, in other words it is important to train all of your muscles in one week, whether it being one, two, three, four, five, six and seven days in the week that you could train you will make progress because I have workouts that will fit everyone's schedule.

Consistency is extremely important as well as keeping it fun because both will guarantee you success! This chapter deals with the various workouts that can be done while on the beach, in the airport waiting for a flight, in a hotel room and anywhere else you can think of while you are having a good time on vacation, or any other party or "good time Charlie" atmosphere. It's so important to train before a party, nightclub because this makes you go out with an advantage of confidence, and a much happier mood. Whenever going out for some nightlife I often try to workout and shower right before. The night is so much more enjoyable this way because your exercise endorphins are giving you that "runners high" which is the greatest "high" ever. The "runners high" not only feels the best but there are no negative drawbacks either, such as DUI's and or negative health side effects being physical or psychological such as depression or anxiety. Any type of drug, alcohol or even lack of sleep will cause you to be depressed the following day, this is a terrible feeling however the "runners high" which is that great feeling induced by exercise causes none of the negative side effects once the "high" wears off as do the other drugs and alcohol. Once your runners high wears off you feel fine, no depression or no anxiety.

Therefore let me stress to you that quality training is extremely important. You will not enjoy the pleasures if the business part is not taken care of and business of course means exercise!

Chapter 3: Different Workouts for Different Places

Wherever you may be: at a party, lounge, night club, cruise, or any other "good time Charlie" situation you must exercise prior to going out or during while on your vacation. Exercise is a priority so make the sacrifices necessary to be able to get that workout in.

Let's see examples of exercise routines that are tailor made for your fun activity.

Let's start with going on a cruise. Most cruises have a full scale gym so chances are that you can go to that gym everyday, say five days of training. Training daily will not only tighten your body and put you in a happier mood so you have a better time on the cruise but it will lessen the hangovers from the previous night's fun or the sea sickness you may experience.

Now not every cruise ship has a gym because I have taken a two day cruise from Venice Italy to Corfu Greece and a three day cruise from Cyprus to Egypt and Israel and sure enough there were no gyms or fitness rooms however they did have a pool but one without water, they must have forgotten to fill it. Luckily no diving attempts were made by any evening goers looking for a
midnight swim!

During that three day "cruise" I had no choice but to invent my own training routine without weights or a pool! Years later I was on a two day cruise from Venice Italy to the island of Corfu, Greece and the same happened, no gym but this ship had a pool which they filled for a few hours per day. During this cruise I ended up doing pull-ups using a rooftop, will explain more later. Nevertheless good workouts were accomplished each time.

This following workout is what I followed myself during a twelve day cruise throughout the Caribbean. We visited ten islands, had a great time filled with great memories and being in shape only added to those memories. Being in shape not only gave me the added energy for sightseeing and hiking on the islands but you would be surprised how many "doors open" for you when your sporting a "build" (an in shape body). It's like an instant friend maker. People either ask you questions about what I eat, how I train, what's my profession, tips they can use, for them a friend, etc. People of all ages seem interested in you when you have a "build". Tour guides even sometimes offer you better prices, etc. People overall appreciate your uniqueness and end up gravitating towards you. However it is extremely important to remain completely humble when you have a "build" because it's so much more appreciated from everyone. Think of a very wealthy person. Isn't it so much more endearing when a wealthy person carries himself in a humble manner as if you had no idea of their fortune? Of course! Now that same wealthy person would not be appreciated if they were a braggart or show off. Yes, now think of the "build" a muscular man or a beautiful woman who either bullies people to get his way or she uses her looks as her primary identity? They would have very few fans to say the least! So let's not forget that humility serves best!

So, having that lean and toned body will most definitely open doors in many places, from the girls appreciating your "build" by the female bartender serving a little more rum in your rum punch or the bouncer letting you skip the line and cover charge in exchange for a few diet/workout tips (that are rarely followed unfortunately). The lean and toned body works great with bouncers and I would sometimes go the extra mile by offering them any assistance in "removing noncompliant" customers. At six foot tall and 205 pounds I am not a giant but I was a New York Golden Gloves boxer and a Two-Time NCAA College All-American wrestler and am an MMA fighter. All of this would facilitate the removal of "noncompliant" customers of a nightclub or lounge. Rarely has my assistance been needed and I am grateful for this because I am a great negotiator and would much rather talks over problems. Remember, humility is key! Nevertheless the nightclub security would greatly appreciate my gesture.

CRUISE SHIP WORKOUT

ADVANCED

A) (If there is a gym): 1 Week Cruise

Monday

Chest

5 sets incline dumbbell press 10-15 reps

5 sets pushups 20-30 reps

5 sets dips 10-15 reps

5 sets pec deck 15-20 reps

Abs

Sit-ups 100 reps

Tuesday

Back

5 sets close grip chin-ups 8-12 reps

5 sets dumbbell rows 8-12 reps

5 sets wide grip pull downs 10-12 reps

5 sets seated cable row 10-12 reps

Wednesday

Biceps, triceps

Superset

5 sets dumbbell curl with 5 sets lying triceps extension 12 reps

5 sets straight bar curls with 5 sets cable pushdowns 15 reps
5 sets preacher curl with 5 sets triceps kickbacks 12 reps

Abs
Leg raises 100 reps

Thursday
Shoulders
5 sets military press 10 reps
5 sets dumbbell lateral raises 15 reps
5 sets upright rows 12 reps
5 sets bent over dumbbell raises 12 reps

Friday
Legs
5 sets walking lunges 20 yards
5 sets stiff legged dead lifts 10 reps
5 sets barbell squats 12 reps
3 sets hack squats 12 reps
3 sets leg curls 12 reps
5 sets calf raises 20 reps

This advanced workout is quite difficult to say the least, taking from thirty to forty-five minutes to complete. Next is the intermediate workout that should take anywhere from twenty-five to forty minutes to complete.

INTERMEDIATE

Monday
Chest, back
Superset

5 sets lat machine pull downs with 5 sets incline bench press 12 reps

5 sets close grip chin-ups with 5 sets dumbbell press 12 reps

5 sets t-bar rows with 5 sets pec-deck

Abs

Crunches 100 reps

Wednesday

Shoulders, biceps triceps

Superset

3 sets dumbbell lateral raises, dumbbell curls and triceps cable pushdowns 12 reps

3 sets upright rows, cable bicep curls, dumbbell triceps extension 12 reps

3 sets reverse peck-deck machine, preacher curls, reverse triceps pushdowns 12 reps

3 sets military press, seated dumbbell curls, triceps kickbacks 12 reps

Abs

Reverse crunches 100 reps

Friday

Legs

Superset

3 sets leg extension with leg curls 20 reps

3 sets hack squats, standing leg curls 15 reps

5 sets walking lunges 20 yards

5 sets calf raises 20 reps

The intermediate involved a lot of super setting which is great for a cardio workout as well. The beginner workout should take between twenty to thirty-five minutes to complete.

BEGINNER

Monday
Upper Body
Superset
5 sets pushups and chin ups 8-12 reps
5 sets dips and pull-ups 8-12 reps
Crunches 50 reps

Thursday
Lower Body
Superset
5 sets leg extension with lying leg curls 15 reps
5 sets barbell squats with stiff legged dead lifts 15 reps
Leg raises 50 reps

The beginner workout is a quick routine that will provide you with the mood enhancing jumpstart that will brighten your day as well as tone your body. Soon enough you will most likely want to move up to the intermediate workout, this is entirely up to you.

Cruise Ship Dining
Large cruise ships often carry thousands of people. Having to feed all of these people is both time consuming and expensive. Lean high protein and high fiber meals are more time consuming and expensive to prepare so sure enough the cruise ship meal plan's priority is not for you to build or maintain a great body. Once again I have taken three cruises and the experience was enhanced times ten because I had a decent physique and it just made the trips that much better. You will see for yourself! Cruise ships pretty much have food available each day from morning until evening and if carefully selected you can eat fairly good meals throughout the day.

Cruise ships often dock for the entire day on little islands or ports allowing you to see for the day a new place. I would always bring food with me so I had extra food to last during the sightseeing, etc. In this chapter I will teach you how to carefully choose your meals that will give you that great body and teach you how to order room service and pack the food for your daily island trip.

Packing food to bring with you when you leave the cruise ship is great because it allows you to save money and eat much leaner. Eating on island restaurants will be more expensive, time consuming and overall less healthy. These restaurants can make your six-pack disappear in two days! Now your vacation just got worse! So, let's not have that happen!

MENU

Breakfast 7 A.M.
4 hard boiled egg whites, 1 whole egg
Fresh fruit
Coffee, tea, water

Also carry out of the cruise ship dining room the same meal of 4 egg whites, 1 whole egg, and fresh fruit. The dining staff will pack the food for you. This meal can be eaten at around 10 a.m.

Lunch 1 P.M.
Grilled chicken breast
Vegetables
Salad (olive oil, vinegar, no salt)

Also carry out sliced turkey breast and 1 whole fruit. This will be your 4 p.m. snack.

Dinner 7 P.M.

1 Glass red/white wine

Broiled fish (ask for it dry, no salt, with lemon)

Salad, vegetables

1 cup fresh fruit

Now if you're docking for the day on an island make sure you pack three extra meals at breakfast so you can eat properly throughout the day on the beach or sightseeing. This type of eating will definitely assist your body towards achieving the leanness that you want, and the added energy you will need to really get the most from this vacation. A good vacation becomes a great vacation when you have the lean and toned body and the increased energy level. Twice I have taken cruises that did not have a gym, one of these "cruises" was a two day ferry ride from Venice, Italy to the island of Corfu, Greece. Never will I forget this magnificent ride down the Adriatic Sea passing through Italy, Slovenia, Croatia, Montenegro, Albania and Greece. Memories that will last a lifetime. Trust me when I say this but the memories were enhanced from the endorphin high I would get from working out and from sporting an in shape physique, that alone speaks for itself. Being one of only two people in great shape on the entire boat is just another added benefit because uniqueness is always appreciated.

The other in shape physique was my friend Eric Lagra, a "good time Charlie" himself. We have taken many trips and will take many more because we have a lot in common, both of us love traveling, training and nightlife! Nevertheless this two day ferry ride didn't have a gym but it did have a pool that was actually filled for a few hours a day, that's better than the Cyprus, Egypt and Israel cruise that forgot to fill the pool with water. I knew something was odd when I saw no lifeguards even though most people in these cultures wear bikini Speedos however sporting a protruding stomach and twelve inch arms was usually a dead give a way that they weren't lifeguards. This two day ferry ride down the Adriatic Sea was nothing short of spectacular while passing every country was amazing and Albania was different due to its vast area of dryness or vegetation, it definitely looked like the hermit s to share a four person cabin with two other people, two truck drivers from Greece who were two great guys but both were smokers and one very overweight which equates to loud snoring. I was able to counteract the snoring by shaking the man in his sleep, he would quickly wake up but I acted as if I was sleeping until he eventually caught me then I told him that my actions wouldn't change and we both agreed.

The first day consisted of lower body the second day upper body exercises. Both done on the top deck with great sunshine and views of the former Yugoslav nation.

2 DAY TOP DECK FERRY BOAT WORKOUT ROUTINE

ADVANCED

Day 1
Legs
12 sets free body squats 20 reps
12 sets walking lunges 20 yards

Abs
Sit-ups 150 reps

Cardio
Deck sprints 5 sprints

Day 2
Upper Body
Superset
Pushups with pull-ups 8 sets
Dips with chin ups 8 sets

Calf raises 300 reps
Leg raises 100 reps
Deck sprints 5 sprints

INTERMEDIATE

Day 1
Full Body
Super Setting 6 sets
Pushups
Pull-ups (wide grip)
Indian push ups
Lunges
Single leg squats
Crunches 100 reps
Deck sprints 10 sprints

Day 2
Perform the same routine because this routine can be performed daily without over training.

BEGINNER

Day 1 or each and everyday while on the cruise.
Superset 5 sets
Pushups 15 reps
Pull-ups 8-12 reps
Free squats 15 reps
Lunges 20 yards
Sit-ups 30 reps
Deck sprints 5 sprints

The dips were performed on the guardrail where the V is, that's the corner of the guardrail where the two guardrails connect. The pull-ups and chin-ups were performed on the edge of the rooftop of one of the storage sheds on the rooftop. Sprinting really raised my-heart rate to further enhance the workout on a cardiovascular basis as well as achieving that "runners high" I had a great time and work-out. Nevertheless walking around shirtless with a "pump" and the post workout endorphin rush was amazing and walking to the pool area to buy a diet soda was the icing on the cake because of a few "turning heads" I received. That's a vacation! Looking good, filled with energy and traveling!

We soon docked in Corfu and what a spectacular island it was! Then stopping in, Montenegro, Croatia, Bosnia, Portugal and Spain. All priceless memories that a large part of I owe to the "build," meaning that traveling with an in shape body made the world of a difference especially abroad which makes you even more unique because they are not used to seeing these physiques even though I must admit that Montenegro really impressed me! Men and women there were incred-ible physical specimens. They were tall, the men were muscular and the women were nicely curved and they were both extremely humble which was an added plus.

Quickly I made friends with the lifeguards, playing water polo and jumping off cliffs into the Adriatic Sea with them. Truly spectacular and it all wouldn't have been possible if it weren't for the decent shape that I was in!

Remember that vacations are for improving or maintaining your body and not abusing it or else you will end up like the typical out of shape person who goes on vacation and is kind of miserable exposing their body on the beach. These out of shape people are more inclined to pass their vacation excessively drinking alcohol and or drugs in order to tell their friends about the trip and how "wasted" they were that they don't even remember a thing! The truth is that they do remember viv-idly but their trip would have been too uneventful and nobody would want to hear about it. It all comes down to action, this is what everyone likes and to provide the action you need a lot of positive energy and this positive energy is definitely created by having a well-toned body, being in shape, and confident. When you arrive to a vacation and cruise ship having a toned body then chanced are that you will exude a positive energy that everyone wants a part of, it's like being the "life of the party". This is why it is so important to maintain your shape or get in shape while on vacation, it's guaranteed just a better time! In my past I have arrived on vacation looking lean and in shape than due to my lack of discipline I would begin slacking off on my diet and workouts and all of a sudden three to four days later I am not looking nearly as sharp as when I arrived. It's a lousy feeling because not only do you feel sluggish from improper eating but it's an awful feeling to notice that less people are "checking you out" and treating you like a regular "Joe Shmo" not asking you about diet tips, workouts, getting that extra smile from whoever you deal with. A great example of this was on a Saturday I won first place at the "East Coast" bodybuilding championship as a light heavy weight competing at 198 pounds. I was in great shape, under five percent body fat!

Then the following day my girlfriend at the time and I flew to Margarita Island, Venezuela. A beautiful Hilton resort with spectacular accommodations. The arrival was great and even better because I was arriving in tip top shape, twenty six years old , at the top of my game, a great physique, money in my pocket, a beautiful woman, nothing could be better! Being there was the ultimate vacation and coming right off a bodybuilding competition my body was very lean but from being on an extremely strict diet for two months I was craving food, big time! Each day there we took boat trips, plane trips, sightseeing, hiking, everyday there was an event and I was up for all of it because of my great shape. During all of these events not a day past that somebody didn't give me either a compliment on my physique or ask me for diet or workout tips.

Walking through crowds, heads turning and that extra smile from the women was all so much fun while it lasted. Then, as the days were passing I was eating the wrong foods and not training which really began affecting me in a negative way. Within days my clothing barely fit, I was feeling very sluggish and less people were even noticing me let alone compliment me. I began vacationing like your average person, drinking too much, overly eating, feeling sloppy and terrible, embarrassed of my body, all combined I became miserable! How it really took that extra fun out of it. The vacation was still great but had I maintained my shape it would've been much better. By the last day I felt like a beached whale while lying by the pool. After a weeks vacation week we were back and the first thing I did was weigh myself to see and I weight 227 pounds! I gained nearly thirty pounds in one week! Going from a six pack to belly, from chiseled jaw line

to round, bloated face! These changes were terrible and never would I allow this to happen again! A good lesson was learned because I lost that edge.

Now back to the cruise ship workouts to further explain that of the three cruises I was on my last one was just a two day ferry ride from Venice Italy to Corfu Greece which I already showed you the way I trained but now I will explain how we ate while on board. Prior to my departure from the U.S.A. I purchased a three pound container of whey protein isolate to bring with me, I poured the contents into a large zip lock bag. It's a great, quick zero carbohydrate meal that will keep your body right for the trip. Five to six ounce pouches of tuna are very convenient also because they are compact and light. Whenever I am traveling or backpacking through a different country I always pack with me the whey protein isolate and sometimes pouches of salmon or tuna. My preference is whey protein isolate because it is more compact that the tuna and the Isopure brand mixes very easily and one and a half scoops in water is all that's needed. Another method I use when traveling abroad is eating fresh vegetables while drinking the whey protein powder. Fresh bottled water, whey protein isolate and vegetables and you are set with a complete and lean meal and with minimal chance of getting sick. Getting sick is very common when traveling abroad and this must be avoided because any sickness will hinder your trip tremendously. We can minimize your chances of getting sick by minimizing eating from food vendors and restaurants. It is very tempting to eat from food vendors because often the scent is tempting and the price is right but it can turn out quite costly to your health and fun on your vacation. Later in this book I will explain more food options regardless of the country you are in.

HOTEL ROOM EXERCISE ROUTINE

Many upscale hotels have decent fitness centers that offer enough exercise equipment to have a sufficient workout and remember a great way to start the day is after drinking a cup of coffee then head over to the fitness center and when your finished training go right ahead and enjoy the free continental breakfast of hard boiled egg whites, fruit and oatmeal. Unfortunately many mid range to more economical hotels such as hostels do not offer any type of fitness centers.

However I often stay in economical hostels and sure enough there is often a gym or YMCA right in the immediate area so make sure to inquire about nearby gyms to your hotel staff if your hotel has no gym. Now, if your hotel has no gym nor is there a local gym in the area I will teach you how to exercise your body to keep up your body and or build up your body for the vacation.

These workouts can either be performed in an outdoor public park and or right in your hotel room.

Let's start with the "hotel room workout". This workout can be performed either twice per week or everyday. I much rather everyday because the "rush" I get from training will last me a few hours which helps me maximize my day. I am just much happier for those few hours so whatever task I do in that time is much more enjoyable! That post workout "high" should always be our goal and motivation for training, its really an incredible feeling, its kind of like that feeling you would get if you received a promotion at work, or won a small lottery, or if you're a guy and you just got that beautiful girls phone number or if you're a girl that cute guy you always liked just asked you out! These are all great and natural feelings that you can feel on a daily basis right after a good hard workout! Me personally, I "Live for this high!" working out before hitting the nightlife further enhances your evening too, later in this book I will teach you how to go out and party with the post workout high and maybe even with a few drinks as well if more ammunition is needed to enhance your nightlife of bars, clubs and dancing!

HOTEL ROOM WORKOUT

ADVANCED

1 Day Full Body Workout
Superset
15 sets, free squats, dips, pull-ups 15 reps
Crunches 100 reps

The dips are performed using either two chairs facing backwards with a two feet separation or on the room balcony in the corner where the balcony hand rails connect perpendicular which looks like a V. The pull-ups are performed either using the hotel rooms' shower curtain rod or holding the top of an open door and lifting your body.

INTERMEDIATE

Superset
10 sets walking lunges, pushups, pull-ups 10 reps (pushups 20 reps)
Crunches 75 reps

BEGINNER
Superset
5 sets, free squats, pull-ups, pushups 10 reps
Crunches 50 reps

All three of these workouts will provide you with a full body workout with cardio included because the supersets increase your heart rate giving you the cardiovascular benefits you will need to further improve your body and health. Hotel rooms vary quite a bit and the most challenging part of a hotel room workout is often the "pull-up" bar and space. Shower curtain rods are often too frail to hold your body weight and using the door for pull-ups isn't easy either so you may have to find another place to perform pull-ups, any bar, ceiling pipe or staircase will usually work fine.

Next I will show you a two day full body workout because I myself rather train my body in two separate days giving me more rest and time to train. One day I will train upper body and the other day lower body. Let me show you.

ADVANCED HOTEL ROOM

(2 day Full Body exercise routine): Day 1
Lower Body
Superset
10 sets free squats, lunges, calf raises 20 reps
Leg raises 100 reps

Day 2
Upper Body
Superset
15 sets pull-ups, dips, Indian pushups 20 reps

INTERMEDIATE

Day 1
Lower Body
Superset
10 reps free squats, lunges, calf raises
Leg raises 75 reps

Day 2
Upper Body
Superset
10 sets pull-ups, dips 15 reps

BEGINNER

Day 1
Upper Body
5 Sets pull-ups 8 reps
5 Sets pushups 10 reps

Day 2
Lower Body
5 sets free squats 12 reps
5 sets lunges 20 yards
Crunches 50 reps

Hotel room workouts can sometimes feel cramped because some hotel rooms are small so to counter this I have often performed lunges and other exercises in the hallway. These hallways are usually not busy with people which enables you to have a better workout. Remember that these "clandestine" workouts can be performed in other areas of the hotel such as pool area, staircase and laundry room (I have performed dips using two washing machines and pushups with my feet on top of the washing machine and my hands on the floor making this almost like an incline bench press!). The main point is that you can workout anywhere whether it being a hotel, park, hallway or even a parking lot you can even use a tree branch for pull-ups! Nothing beats the feeling of working out in your hotel room then showering and then heading out to tackle your day or evening with so much more enthusiasm. Talk about a great way to eliminate jet lag and anxiety a workout with effectively treat jet lag, anxiety, depression and a hangover, naturally. Sweating is definitely an effective treatment for anyone.

Chapter 4: Eating and Training Abroad

Traveling abroad is a lot of fun for me. Most all of it is a great experience especially eating the local cuisine. This however can cause havoc on your body, both your appearance and your health. Being in a completely new environment can have an adverse effect on your body. These adverse effects could be water retention, sleep pattern disorders, diarrhea, headache and upset stomach. Any of these symptoms can ruin your vacation to say the least.

Even the slightest symptoms such as water retention can take a great body and turn it into to just an average body and now with that average body your vacation now dropped a lot of points unless your vacation in skiing somewhere and even then having a boated face will ruin your nightlife and chances of meeting someone that night! Our only option is to minimize the chances of getting sick while on vacation abroad.

So how do we do this? By eating right. Definitely while abroad sample the local cuisine but keep it to a minimum by eating small portions. While abroad I always sample the local cuisine but I do this by taking a bite or two then giving the rest to a stray animal or throwing it out. This works great because I get to taste the food but with minimal calories and chances of getting sick. It's like having the best of both worlds! Traveling isn't easy and is very tiring so not training and eating properly will take its toll on you by making you even more tired. Stopping at local vegetable and fruit stands to eat vegetables is a great option along with a can of tuna in water that can easily be purchased anywhere. Tuna and vegetables really make a great meal except that a pretty waitress won't be serving you, the only real advantage of eating out! For example, a vegetable and tuna meal will cost you maybe two or three dollars at most (except if your in western Europe) , provide a great meal, and you will save so much more time than eating out so now you will have more time to enjoy your vacation and more money too! Eating with street vendors can be risky therefore you may become sick.

If you choose to eat with a street vendor be careful and try to eat plain chicken breast or grilled fish and corn. Hotels offer decent restaurants but usually at a premium. Another tactic I use when traveling abroad is whey protein isolate powder. Before a trip I bring a three pound container of "Isopure" and pour the contents into a double lined zip lock plastic bag. This works great because whenever I am hungry I simply open the zip lock bag pour one and a half scoops of whey into a cup and mix with water, usually only bottled water when I am abroad. That's a great "leaning out" meal because it's straight protein with no carbs or fat.

If this meal is not enough for you then add a few raw vegetables or fruit. You can eat this every two to four hours and see yourself "lean out" as the day or days go on, it's a great feeling to be on top of your game while abroad on vacation.

Exercising abroad is rather simple because you may find a gym or if not then a park or hotel room will work fine and training on the beach is a lot of fun too! What better way is there to show off your "build" than on the beach! Country to country lifestyles and cultures change dramatically. Training, diet, nightlife, sightseeing, etc. You must train and eat right everywhere regardless of the country you are in. Some countries are more difficult than others. I will share with you a few of my experiences in different countries on how I kept in shape. I will start off with the continuation of the wonderful cruise my friend Eric and I took from Venice Italy to Corfu Greece. We took a twelve day trip which began with the "running of the bulls" in Pamplona, Spain and what a great time that was!

PAMPLONA, SPAIN, RUNNING OF THE BULLS

We arrived in Madrid then connected with a magnificent high speed train ride to Pamplona. During that train ride we drank the whey protein isolate along with a few diet sodas because we needed the caffeine boost being that we were so jet lagged from the New York to Madrid flight that was already seven hours delayed and we were exhausted. I am not a total caffeine fan because has its negative aspects such as the release of cortisol which is a stress hormone.

Once arrived to Pamplona we checked into the hotel and rested for a while before hitting the nightlife. I didn't workout that day due to exhaustion but I ate grilled fish and a salad for dinner and for a treat some fried "Churros" (fried doe). It's fine to cheat a little on your diet because we must not forget that A) we are human, B) this type of healthy lifestyle is like a marathon meaning it's for the long haul so choose a pace that you can sustain fairly easily.

That evening we went to the bar district. Beautiful old buildings and cobblestone streets packed with people drinking, dancing and having fun. One thing about Spain is that the people dress extremely well which makes the nightlife that much nicer. Drinking alcohol and getting in shape may not be the best combination but you can still do it. Why live a boring life? Who doesn't like to party? For a long time I went out on the party scene completely sober and yes it was fun but it became a little more fun with a small amount of alcohol to feel a bit looser. Being completely sober when other people aren't usually equals no fun.

Anyway we started off the evening with a "Kalimocha" which is red wine mixed with Pepsi but we had it with diet Pepsi. Two of those were all that was needed to enjoy the evening with minimal calories consumed. The next morning we ran with the bulls (sober) and had an awesome time! What a rush! Then we all went to the arena that was packed with wild bulls and hundreds of people all teasing and running away from the bulls. I fell a few times chasing and running from these bulls. An experience of a lifetime! That evening we boarded the high speed train to Madrid where we spent a grueling night in a non air conditioned hostel with no breeze either, a long night that was because it was ninety seven degrees in Madrid. The next morning we boarded a flight to Venice Italy. During that entire day we exercised with pull-ups and pushups at a park and ate a lot of vegetables, fruit, tuna and whey protein. This kept us in shape which is exactly the goal on vacation, styling!

VENICE, ITALY

This was a rather short trip, just a day to sightsee the beautiful and historic city. While walking through the city I drank an espresso coffee to help suppress my appetite and a gelato but unfortunately they didn't have sugar free. We walked the city while waiting for our boat ride to Corfu, Greece. Italy has a special flare to it, the way people dress and carry themselves is a lot to be said. Being that my family is all Spaniard which is a similar culture to Italy has taught me a lot about the divine Western European culture which quality of life is their top priority.

Venice was very hot that day so we took off the day of training because I would train that evening on the boat. Eating in Venice could be calorie laden but I chose to only cheat on my diet a little with the gelato. After a day of sightseeing Venice we then boarded the tremendous ferry to Corfu Greece.

Venice Meals

Broiled grouper with lemon
Salad, vegetables
Sugar-free Italian ice

FERRY RIDE TO CORFU, GREECE

Again, this was another day trip on route up the Adriatic Coast and our next stop would be another ferry ride to mainland Greece. Corfu and the entire Greek culture is among my favorites in the world. The climate is great and so is the cuisine, very healthy for being in shape because Greeks don't usually fry their food but they BBQ it instead which is much healthier. Greece is perfect for a fitness nut like me because the food is tasty yet healthy and the weather is warm enough to have your shirt off to show the results of a healthy lifestyle. Very attractive Mediterranean people I must add though not as well dressed as Italy or Spain but Greeks have great olive toned skin. A quiet Island but picturesque to say the least. I was able to eat healthy, train and finish off with a shot of Ouzo which is their national after dinner liquor.

CORFU DIET

Greek Meals

1) BBQ Octopus
Greek salad
Shot of Ouzo

2) BBQ whole Red Snapper with olive oil and lemon
Cucumber, tomato Greek salad
Glass white wine

Training in Corfu just consisted of walking with backpacks all over the island. The calisthenics workout was put off until that evening when we would be spending the next two nights in . That late afternoon we boarded the short ferry ride to mainland Greece where we had a taxi drop us off at the Albanian border. The taxi was not allowed to cross the border so we left the taxi ten yards from the border and we walked across into Albania. Customs stamped our passports then after walking a little to find a taxi we asked to be driven to Saranda Beach, an Albanian vacation spot.

Albania certainly was different as if time stopped fifty years ago which is kind of cool and mysterious if you ask me! Driving a few hours to Saranda wasn't easy because the roads were barely paved, bumpy and narrow. The roads weren't really built for cars. In 1992 Albania had 2,000 cars, mainly government vehicles and today there are around 700,000! There were concrete gun tower bunkers all over the roadside.

Once arriving to Saranda we settled in a nice hotel that was only thirty five dollars per night with breakfast included. After checking in I drank the whey powder and ate an apple then we knew we had to work out. Here is how I trained:

Saranda Beach, Albania Workout

Walking on the beach I found a park so the swing set made for a great pull-up bar and pushups and free squats were performed on the sand.

10 sets
Supersetted
Pull-ups 12 reps
Indian pushups 12 reps
Pushups 25 reps
Free squats 25 reps

An excellent workout and the entire time overlooking the view of the Adriatic Sea and listening to a man playing the violin on the board-walk. Feeling the sweat and adrenaline only improved the moment! I wouldn't trade that workout for a Gold's Gym workout ever! The workout was definitely an awesome prerequisite for an evening of fun in the Albanian nightlife of dancing, drinking and fun.

After a good workout you are feeling unbelievable on the " high" for at least an hour or two and training as we did an hour before hit-ting the scene only added to the fun, feeling great, looking athletic so what could be better? Actually a drink or two of straight vodka, rum or gin provides that slight boost and mellow feeling all at the same time making you have a terrific evening of talking, dancing, flirting, etc. When you're a done training your metabolism is racing so any small amount of alcohol will simply rush into your system which doubles the effect of the drink, so the good news is that you will feel the buzz with fewer drinks which means fewer calories so your physique will stay intact. It worked great for me! A workout, shower then a drink or two at a club and that's a recipe for fun! I highly recommend it (AA members not included).

Nevertheless the nightlife in Saranda went from good to great and being a foreigner adds to your appeal and having a nice physique adds *way* more appeal! (Dressing poorly will destroy this
package!) The clubs were interesting but for being in an evening in July they were not that crowded. Nevertheless it was a great evening thanks largely to the confident feeling you have when you're in shape. One of the many times when you notice the sacrifices you made were one hundred percent worth it.

Drinking Alcohol
Drink and have fun with less calories and hangover

Drinking only one or two drinks is all you need to feel the benefits because when you are in shape and eating clean your body will easily respond to minimal alcohol and your body will respond with needing even less alcohol if you drink immediately following a workout because your metabolism is really racing in high gear. Obviously it's always better to drink less alcohol because your sleep will be better because any drug or alcohol will hinder your deep REM sleep (the sleep that really counts). REM sleep is so important because that is when your body repairs itself and produces its own natural HGH and HGH production is crucial for so maintaining youth, burn body fat, skin elasticity, vision, and a number of other positive benefits. Good sleep equals thirty three percent of your success in creating an incredible body, the other sixty six percent is thirty three percent nutrition and thirty three working out. For an example think of a camera that's standing on a tripod.

So what would happen to the camera if one of the legs of the tripod was removed or broken? The camera would fall because all three legs of the tripod are equally important for keeping the camera up without falling. Now think of the tripod and the success of creating your nice body which is thirty three percent eating right, thirty three percent rest and thirty three training, all equally important to creating the body you want! Makes sense, right!

Now back to drinking alcohol which of course anything more than three ounces of wine isn't that healthy but then again what the heck! We all deserve to get a little crazy and loosen up a bit! Drinking small amounts of the right alcohol will barely hurt your physique and the minimal hangover will be treated effectively by exercising in the morning. Definitely stay clear away from your fancy drinks such as Margaritas, Mojitos, Pina Coladas, frozen daiquiris, etc. Drinking vodka, whiskey, gin, rum, and wine are good bets if they are prepared straight, on the rocks, or with diet soda or club soda. Drinks prepared this way will have minimal calories that will help you avoid getting that sloppy physique. Remember that trips are much more enjoyable when you are partying a little and IN SHAPE as opposed to the norm of partying too much and be OUT OF SHAPE!

Best Choices for Drinking Alcohol
Gin

Vodka

Whiskey

Scotch

Tequila

Rum (use less of the 151 proof)

Everclear (be extremely careful due to its 190 proof of alcohol)

Aguardiente of Spain (the clear Aguardiente has less sugar and more alcohol potency)

Wine, either red or white (wine does not have much alcohol concentration but it has numerous health benefits)

All of these are to be prepared either straight, on the rocks or mixed with diet soda. It is extremely important to drink plenty of water while you are out on a night of drinking and partying because this will minimize the hangover because alcohol is a diuretic and dehydration will cause havoc to your body so drink at least a quart of water when you are dinking alcohol.

Finishing off at Saranda Beach

After a great time in Saranda Beach we finished off the day meeting a few ballerina dancers from Romania that were there to perform in an event. Pleasant people so we all hung out on the beach which was quite pebbly and the Adriatic Sea was a comfortable maybe seventy six degrees. We had told the performers that we were taking a taxi to Tirana, the country's capital. They weren't familiar with Tirana but when we told them that after a night in Tirana we would be off to Montenegro the following morning and all of a sudden their eyes lit up when I mentioned "Montenegro" and quickly they responded "Budva Beach"! Budva Beach was THE place in Montenegro they said also Major US celebrities such as Madonna recently purchased vacation properties there. Now we new where to go in Montenegro and were excited about it!

That late afternoon I ran three to four miles enabling me to see the scenery. Albania was totally different from any other western European country in every way. After the run I stopped at a small grocery store and purchased a liter of water, a can of tuna in water, an apple and a raw cucumber. This was the ideal post workout meal for even a better price too! Actually I purchased a few more tunas , water and vegetables to bring along on the five hour taxi ride to Tirana that we were about to begin.

Eating and Training that Day in Saranda Beach

Hotel Breakfast
5 hard boiled egg whites and 1 whole hard boiled egg
Fresh fruit
Coffee with skim milk no sugar, 2 glasses of water

Snack
1 ½ scoop whey powder mixed with water, 1 apple
Lunch (street vendor)
1 BBQ chicken and vegetable skewer

Snack
BBQ shrimp and vegetable

Dinner
Broiled Sturgeon fish with lime and olives
Cucumber salad
Vegetables (squash)

Saranda Beach Workout

This was a simple four mile run through the streets, boardwalk and beach. Running on the beach is much more tiring but it's a much better workout than running on pavement and much easier on your joints too. After the run the feeling was great and a great prerequisite for the five hour taxi ride we were about to take to Tirana. A good workout works wonders for anxiety.

Post Workout Meal
Orange
Raw squash
Can of mackerel in water

TIRANA, ALBANIA: LONG RIDE, DANGEROUS EVENING

Riding in a taxi through Albania was not easy but quite picturesque. The roads were narrow and littering didn't seem offensive. Stopping several times to take pictures of the landscape and the numerous concrete war bunkers that were all over the roadside. The vast mountains and hills were beautiful and seizing the moment was the secret. When could I ever backpack up the Adriatic coastline with a good friend, in shape and free as a bird! You realize that life is short, youth is even shorter and at the end of the day we are only left with memories! Right! So why not make as many memories as we can! During the long and bumpy ride we stopped at a restaurant to eat lamb and cucumber salad. This restaurant was in the middle of nowhere but this only added to the appeal. Having a few muscles definitely makes you unique but in the U.S. you will see people that are lean and toned from time to time but in Albania? Never! So the restaurant staff was pleased to have us there, asking for pictures, making a muscle for them and even a few arm wrestling matches. A tasty Albanian healthy meal and most of all another wonderful memory that will last a lifetime! Away we were back in the taxi half way on our way to Tirana.

Two hours later we stopped to eat the food I had packed with me which was tuna, vegetables and a half liter of water. It doesn't sound tasty because it wasn't but when you know the meal is improving your body then all of a sudden you're more pleased especially when you are finished because you won't feel guilty after eating the wrong foods nor will you feel bloated. Finally arriving in Tirana and how evident it was due to the city lights that were noticed kilometers away and as we came closer the pollution smog over the city was evident as well. The pollution smog combined with ninety-five degree July heat equaled an unpleasant and humid feeling. We checked into a hotel right in the center of town, a nice place especially at sixty dollars for the night. We immediately had some whey powder with water and a fruit.

Earlier that day while in Saranda Beach I had gone for a run which completed the day's workout. With the beach, a workout and healthy eating already out of the way now the only part of the vacation left was a night out in the city of Tirana. Dressing in shorts and flip flops is not the norm pretty much anywhere in Europe so I wore a nice outfit of jeans, shoes and a V-neck silky t-shirt. A great combo when you want to slightly expose your body without looking like a show off. It seems as though women have X-ray vision because regardless of what you are wearing women always know what type of body you have underneath so definitely wearing skin tight clothing is a no no, nobody appreciates a "show off" or "tough guy".

Starting the evening walking through the streets toward the "scene" I was amazed how nicely developed the city was. New buildings, lounges, restaurants and high end boutiques were abound. We stopped at a very nice lounge had a glass of Albanian red wine and enjoyed the ambiance. Europe has amazing décor and architecture and the people always dress so nice not to mention many of the Albanian women have that exotic Mediterranean look. It seems that when your are abroad you can see that the women are extremely feminine and the men perhaps more reserved. Approaching women was an interesting challenge considering the language barrier. I can speak five languages but unfortunately Albanian wasn't one of them. Not speaking Albanian was an obstacle but I soon realized that many Albanians spoke Italian which I spoke fluently so now I was on an "even playing field". If an Albanian didn't speak Italian they may speak some English. Speaking to women at an international level there is always one common denominator that works everywhere and that is good old humor! I may have many weaknesses but a sense of humor was always a big part of my personality. Sure enough a few of the people were laughing either at me or with me but nevertheless they were laughing! That's good enough. Soon we left to go to a nightclub that was recommended by the people we were talking to in the previous lounge. Within walking distance was this extravagant nightclub. Sure enough I kind of felt the red carpet treatment from the bouncer's thanks for my being in shape. Once inside the place was beautiful but all of a sudden things changed for the worse.

TIRANA NIGHTLIFE (NOT TOO SAFE)

Great weather, attractive people, good music and a nice décor are all the tools needed for a good night of fun. Quickly I drank a vodka and club soda. A good drink because of minimal calories but the club soda will rehydrate your body unlike just straight vodka or a diet coke and vodka because the coke has caffeine and that's even another diuretic. Vodkas and orange or cranberry juice isn't wise either because the juices add unwanted sugar and calories. By my second drink, first a glass of red wine at the previous place and now this vodka and club soda I was feeling pretty good but I needed an extra kick so another vodka and club soon followed. Now everything was falling into place and the club now seemed that much better. Then I approached an attractive woman and started making her giggle, we spoke in Italian. Everything was running smooth until we moved closer to a heavily guarded table with several bodyguards guarding it.

Albania is laden with mobsters and it was evident that table was filled with them but little did I know I became to close to the guarded table and to make matters worse the woman I was socializing with was one of their girlfriends or wives, either one is trouble for me. Sure enough one of the bouncers rudely approached me and in Italian he told me to leave the club but being that I didn't appreciate his attitude I quickly responded "no I wont leave, I like it here" I had said it in a manner that showed confidence and innocence because I acted as if he was being polite and I was not one bit intimidated. Things only got worse when several bouncers approached me while one spit on me. I kept my cool and made a fist with one hand and punched my other hand and said lets go outside so we can take care of business. Basically I called him out to fight outside the nightclub one on one. I felt great, maybe a bit tipsy which only meant my fight timing would be slightly off and perhaps I would've absorbed an extra punch or two, overall not an issue for me so beating him up still would've been a walk in the park. So outside I went waiting for a minute or two then practically the entire male population of the nightclub came after me with bottles, sticks, and chairs in their hands. I now realized that I would have to retreat because I had about 1500 dollars in my pocket which would've been taken after I was beaten up and perhaps an evening in an Albanian jail, neither is any fun. Quickly I began running away from the crowd at full speed, thankfully may conditioning was great because a week earlier I had just won an underground MMA fight in Manhattan which I had trained really intense for, so cardio wise I knew this club crowd had nothing on me. After two full blocks all but one of the guys from the club couldn't continue running due to exhaustion yet I was still fresh as a daisy so now two blocks after that the one person that was still chasing me was now becoming exhausted as well. For a minute I was thinking of stopping in order to beat up this lone survivor, this would've been a lot of fun but I then decided not to only because while I would be busy fighting this person up the others may have recuperated and caught up to me. Again the 1500 dollars in my pocket was not worth losing while a few bruises I could deal with but not minus the money because it would be needed for my trip and my heart was set on my next stop, "Budva Beach, Montenegro". Safely I returned to my room then read a little, ate a tuna and apple then went to sleep , another great experience and again thanks to my great shape, this time it didn't work for the ladies but it saved my money and possibly a few broken bones instead. I am not a model nor close to it but I don't want a broken nose, my cauliflower ear from wrestling is bad enough! A great evening nevertheless! At this point we decided to travel further up north along the Adriatic Sea to a more peaceful and safer place even though a little danger and mischief never hurt anybody!

Albania was a great place, quite and interesting too. Montenegro was a simple bus ride and taxi away. The following morning I had arranged for a taxi to take us to the border of Montenegro even though it would be a long and expensive ride, well worth it though. At the border we were dropped off so we walked into Montenegro after clearing customs then we immediately found a taxi that would take us to Budva Beach. Leaving Tirana wasn't easy due to all the traffic and bumpy mountainside roads. Along the ride the taxi stopped at a local restaurant almost in the middle of nowhere but we enjoyed a fantastic meal.

Taxi Ride to Budva Beach, Montenegro

Albania Restaurant Meal
Broiled Steak (Home grown organic)
Zucchini
Salad with olive oil, vinegar and cheese
Liter of water

The delicious and nutritious meal came with a unique ambiance I must admit. Here we are the three of us, the taxi driver, me and Eric. Both Eric and I are in shape so of course having a lean and toned body in a country like Albania is a rarity along with being a tourist. The restaurant staff began practicing their English and asked for some pictures of us, I know that it sounds corny but these people really appreciated it but what was quite surprising was the eighty two year old Grandma that was as strong as an ox because when she shook my hand she nearly broke it! The main thing is that the restaurant meal was healthy allowing me to keep up my shape. A few hours after we arrived at the border with Montenegro but the taxi had to leave us because he wasn't permitted to drive into the new country. That seems to be the norm with these countries because unlike the European Union the countries really aren't combined that way.

Budva Beach, Montenegro

Once arriving in Montenegro on route to Budva Beach it was evident that we had left Albania because Montenegro seemed more modernized and clean. The hills were spectacular and the views of the Adriatic Sea were breath taking. Already having the feeling that we were in some type of paradise because I just had that feeling. Sure enough we arrived at the cliff over Budva Beach to take a few pictures and looking down onto Budva Beach was spectacular. Driving down the winding hill into the small city I began reading my travel book in order to find hotel accommodations. The hotel was beautiful, beachfront and less than one hundred dollars per night, what a steal! I was really excited about this new place and experience because everything just felt perfect. Budva Beach was quite a paradise starting with the best looking people I have ever seen. Women were tall and curvy while the men were six foot four and muscular. Their complexion was somewhat of an olive skin and the hair both blond and brunette. Everyone was in shape sort of like Rio de Janeiro but with even a better vibe. The people were in shape because I quickly noticed that playing sports was a big part of their culture and the food was rather simple, just chicken breast, fish and salad. I cannot stress enough to you the amount of beautiful people that were roaming around, especially the women. I was in awe!

After checking in we quickly had a meal consisting of whey protein isolate and an apple. Nothing like a healthy and lean meal that will keep your six pack in check because with the good looking people roaming around at all times I had to keep my "A" game of being in shape, dressing well and being polite with a sense of humor. After eating I went to the beach to enjoy the atmosphere and exercise while there. Working out on the beach under the bright sunlight isn't easy but it had to be done.

Wearing a baseball cap and sunglasses helps quite a bit along with a white t shirt. Looking to find some type of pull-up bar I noticed that the lifeguards were sitting way up on their chairs, about seven feet high and some type of scaffold was supporting the chairs. The scaffold had numerous bars that would be great for doing pull-ups and "windshield wipers" now all I needed was a type of "dip" bar for my chest workout. I couldn't put together a dip bar so I settled for push-ups, the "old reliable" for a chest, triceps and front deltoid workout.

Day 1 Budva Beach Workout and Meals

Chest, Back, Shoulders, Biceps and Triceps
Pull-ups wide grip with knees raised 6 sets, 12 reps
Push-ups hands wide apart 6 sets 12 reps
Swim "all out" 10-20 yards

All 3 of these exercises are super setted. Ex. pull-up to a push-up to a swim non stop.

Meals

Lunch
1 ½ scoops of Isopure whey protein isolate
1 apple

Late afternoon snack (at a street vendor)
Grilled chicken on pita bread, lettuce and tomato
½ liter of water.

Dinner (at a restaurant)
Red cabbage salad
Grilled Red Snapper fish
Small frozen yogurt
Liter of water

Nightlife
Vodka with club soda
Glass red wine

The first day in Budva Beach was going smoothly due to the fact that the necessities were taken care of first meaning the workout and healthy eating. With that now out of the way the rest of the day was that much better. After the beach I wandered around amazed at the classical European architecture. Europe is filled with amazing architecture, cobblestone streets and history. You are really in another world.

The night came so I dressed up with shoes, jeans and a nice V-neck T-shirt. In Montenegro the people weren't as stylish as either Italy or Spain but they were still dressed nice. No matter where you are in Europe the people usually are well dressed. Budva Beach was loaded with outdoor clubs, restaurant and bars all on the waterfront. It was blistering hot during the day so the evenings were warm which made the outdoor clubs pleasantly comfortable. Drinks were reasonably priced and the women were extremely attractive, a good combination. I quickly ordered and drank a "Stoli" vodka with club soda and fifteen minutes later a glass of red wine.

With the two drinks in my system I felt it was now time to mingle and get to know people. Getting through the language barrier was part of the challenge but nevertheless we met several people and quickly found out more about the scene. Friendly people for sure. Unlike Spain and other parts of Europe the nightlife ended at one in the morning. For us that is quite alright because it meant starting an earlier day on the beach and training the following day. With only two drinks there was no hangover.

Day 2 Budva Beach

Day two began with an early morning three mile jog followed by breakfast at the hotel that was included. The breakfast was a buffet and on that buffet there were few healthy options so I stuck with hard boiled egg whites and fresh fruit with a cup of strong European coffee. All done by ten a.m. What a way to start a beautiful ninety five degree day filled with beautiful people in bathing suits all over the place. Following the morning jog, breakfast and a shower the beach was next. By eleven a.m. it was off to the beach. The beaches there all had lounge chairs, waitresses and nice music. It almost felt like a nightlife atmosphere.

While I was walking on the beach as usual a few looks and glances because I was fit but what surprised me was that the lifeguard approached me to ask me what type of athlete I was so I told him that a week earlier I had just fought and won an MMA fight in NYC.

We immediately got along because he too had a toned physique and was a kick boxer. He was super nice to me and immediately he let me use the lifeguard kayak and paddle boats. Within an hour we were jumping off a fifty foot cliff into the sea. What a rush! Later on we worked out and he showed me some kick boxing moves while I showed him wrestling moves. Within no time I had a crowd of kids asking me to teach them wrestling moves and of course I did willingly. A great day on the beach and after I went to a street vendor and ate a grilled fish on a pita bread with greens and a bottle of water. That evening we went to a few bars to mingle and have fun. The women were so tall. One woman asked me if I was Italian so I answered no I am Spaniard. I asked the tall beautiful woman why she thought I was Italian and she responded "because you are short" that killed my ego! Being the six feet tall that I am I never considered myself to be short but I guess to Montenegrin standards I was, that hurt. Later on going to a nice outdoor club I drank a Bacardi 151 with diet coke and that one drink did the trick because it was twice as powerful as regular rum. With one drink everything was good, the mingling, socializing, etc. what a great night!

Day 2 Budva Beach

Exercise
3 Mile run (early morning)

Meals

Breakfast
5 hard boiled egg white and 1 hard boiled egg

Fresh fruit
Coffee, water

Lunch
Can of light tuna in water
Fruit

Late afternoon snack
Grilled fish on a pita bread
½ liter water

Dinner
Broiled steak
Sautéed vegetables

Nightlife
1 Bacardi "151" rum with diet coke

Day 3 Budva Beach

By the third day I was feeling really comfortable and in a nice routine of training, eating right and having fun. Different cultures always impressed me and Montenegro definitely took me by surprise with its beauty, reasonable prices and not to mention beautiful people. Backpack traveling gets exhausting after a while due to the fact that your routine is" thrown out of wack". In order to minimize being "thrown out of wack" it is necessary to eat right and workout every day. Nevertheless hopping from country to country, hotel to hotel eventually gets to be tiring. This is why staying put in Budva Beach was wonderful because a steady routine of training, dieting and fun happened each day there. Awake by nine a.m. I set off for a short two mile run at a very fast pace with a few sprints during those two miles. This high impact type of cardio is a great natural growth hormone releaser plus the fast pace intensifies the "runner high" that I look for during every workout. Let me tell you that the runners high is the ultimate feeling! Getting that "runners high" is the main reason why I workout everyday, it's an incredible sensation.

After that intense run I went down to the hotel breakfast area to eat. That day I had non fat yogurt, fresh fruit and an egg white and vegetable omelet with a cup of tea and water. Nothing beats the feeling of a healthy meal following a nice workout. The rest of the day would be relaxing until the evening weight training workout. Right after a nice warm shower I was off to the beach.

While walking on the beach a few women asked me if my friend Eric and I were from the "States" of course we responded "yes". The women told us that they figured we were American because we were in good shape. Of course that was a tremendous compliment because America is perhaps the only country where lifting weights and exercising is main stream. Having a lean and toned body opens a lot of doors especially in remote foreign countries like Montenegro. The girls were really cool and not "hustlers" either. A woman who is a "hustler" knows how to take advantage of guys like drinking and eating at the guy's expense in exchange for a few fake compliments and flirting. I avoid "hustlers" at all costs because I feel that my "game" is still "tight" enough to attract normal women and not "hustlers". To keep up your "game" it is crucial to be fit, charming, chivalrous, well groomed, educated and well dressed. The girls we met were very decent women nevertheless. Shortly after because of the "ADD" type of guy I am I decided to leave and go for a kayak ride to the cliff where I was a day before jumping into the pristine Adriatic Sea. As I was leaving I had offered the girls a kayak ride and of course one opted. Let me tell you that women are always spontaneous and up for an adventure at any time! And I'm an adventure, risk taking type of guy! As soon as she boarded I paddled away towards the cliff. As soon as we arrived a dove into the water to climb the cliff to the top and "bam" jump into the sea. What a rush! Loved it so much I went up and jumped three times! The girl patiently waited in the kayak thinking that I was a lunatic for jumping off such a high cliff with no experience, and three times no less! I re-boarded the kayak and began paddling to shore, she loved the fact that I was only rowing because that's just being a gentleman, right. As soon as we came close to shore one of my lifeguard friends snuck up behind us and tipped over the kayak! A nice splash and a lot of fun but I had brought a camera with me and it was ruined, my second broken camera in a week. My first camera broke while in Pamplona Spain when I fell and it smashed in my pocket while I was running away from a bull. That time I didn't mind one bit! Nevertheless we both fell in the water but she and I were both decent swimmers.

After the beach I took a nice walk through the enclosed "Old Town". It's an ancient town that is fully enclosed to protect itself from wars in the past. Very unique little town! That late afternoon I went to the local gym that my lifeguard friend recommended. It was decent and the people were so friendly they didn't even charge Eric and me. One the former NY Knicks basketball player was there and at seven foot five it was obvious. Montenegro was filled with such tall people!

Following a great workout of a full body intense workout I sat in the steam room to relax. That late afternoon we boarded a bus to Croatia, the first stop being Dubrovnik.

Day 3 Budva Beach, Montenegro

Workout
Full body giant set
Squats to leg curls to lat machine pull downs to barbell curls to triceps Push down to military press
5 sets non-stop 8-12 repetitions
All completed within 40 minutes

Meals

Breakfast
Egg white and vegetable omelet
Nonfat sugar free yogurt
Tea, water

Snack
Can of tuna
Cucumber

Lunch
Grilled Salmon with beets

Pre-workout snack
1½ scoop whey protein isolate
1 Orange

Dinner (post workout)
Swordfish Grilled with lemon and pepper
Rice
Turnips and Brussels sprouts

BUS RIDE FROM MONTENEGRO TO CROATIA

Up until this point most of this trip was traveled by taxi, airplane, train and ferry but never bus. Never did I enjoy bus rides as much as the other forms of transportation. When preparing to leave Budva Beach many people had recommended taking the bus to Dubrovnik, Croatia. Even though I agreed it was still against my original choice being taxi. Yes the financial savings were substantial but that's about it. Sure enough upon boarding the bus it was packed for a five hour ride. About an hour into the ride the bus driver tried to evict a few English backpackers because the driver claimed they didn't pay. It turns out that he was just trying to "hustle" them for more money. Seeing the unjust I quickly intervened and defended the backpackers and told the driver to leave them alone because they would not give the driver any more money. I was firm so the driver listened. The girls remained grateful so we all went out that evening once we arrived to Dubrovnik.

However during the trip there would be more turmoil and delays. It turned out that my friend Eric was sitting next to an ex con would was in prison in Montenegro. Upon arrival to the Croatian border they ran all of our passports through their computer and sure enough the ex con was apprehended and the entire bus and our luggage had to be checked. Actually the ex con was a funny guy he had many of us laughing throughout the ride. Hopefully he ended up ok. Finally we arrived and during that five hour ride my two meals consisted of two cans of lump crabmeat and two big pieces of watermelon. Sounds like an odd mix but eating right's priority is nutrition and balance, the crab provided the protein and omega three fats and the watermelon provided the fiber and carbohydrates. It was a good meal with no harm at all to the physique.

Arriving in Dubrovnik was a cool experience, it was midnight, warm and in a new country. After leaving the bus the bus station had a few people offering us rooms for the night and at decent prices as well. For twenty five dollars each me and my travel buddy Eric were hooked up in a nice air conditioned apartment that we shared with a Korean family. It just added to the experience. We then met up with the English backpackers and walked to the downtown nightlife area were all the fun was at. As typical backpackers the three girls were on a budget therefore they initially felt uncomfortable having a few drinks at a nice club. They first tried to buy me a drink for defending them with the bus driver incident but I told them jokingly that I never allow any woman to buy me a drink because then at the end of the night they "expect something in return" and I'm not "easy"! They laughed then I told them not to worry because drinks are on me. This is what I am used to, the man always paying when out with women. After ordering a round for them I ordered lemon vodka with club soda followed by another one. With two drinks I was off to a great time. Nevertheless the backpackers had a great time with us! Definitely a blast! Cobblestone streets, tall stone walls and being in an enclosed city made it more memorable!

These are the two meals that were eaten on the bus ride:

Meal 1
1 Can of lump crabmeat with a piece of watermelon

Meal 2
1 Can of lump crabmeat with a piece of honeydew

Daytime came early and being up at eight a.m. the day was started by a short two mile run followed by an upper body workout that I did on the monkey bars at a park. Pushups, pull-ups and dips, 10 sets of each and I was feeling that nice "runners high". What a great way to start the day!

Immediately after the workout I had breakfast consisting of one nonfat yogurt drink and a piece of fresh bread eaten right at the bakery. Then while walking through the historic city I noticed so many foreign tourists. This was the complete opposite of the pristine Montenegro. After walking through the castles and fort I then started looking for a taxi to go to Split, a port city with boat trips to the Dalmatian coast. Hvar Island was recommended by the girl who fell overboard with me in the kayak in Montenegro. She said that it was the place to go on the Dalmatian coast but I was doubtful that any resort area could top Budva Beach.

Dubrovnik to Split would be a several hour ride and we would get to cross into Bosnia for only about twelve miles on our way to Split. Bosnia is definitely the least popular for tourism than any other country in the former Yugoslavia. Slovenia possibly being the most stabilized country of all of them. On the taxi ride we noticed many beautiful sights of mountains, hills and scattered valleys and lakes.

We stopped several times to take pictures and to buy fresh fruit at a fruit stand. The scenery was spectacular. We soon entered the Bosnian border from Croatia and it was a very quick experience with the border police simply asking our nationality. Bosnia is quite a large country considering the location but unfortunately for Bosnia the coastline is merely about twelve miles.

Crossing into Bosnia I noticed a more perhaps primitive country because I noticed cheaper Russian and Czech made cars and motorcycles and nobody on motorcycle was wearing a helmet, just like in Albania. Surprisingly the shoreline wasn't crowded at all. To me that didn't make any sense because for such a large country the beach front land is minimal so I figured that it would've been overly developed with hotels, tourism and with the homes of the wealthy but I guess I was wrong. The roughly twelve miles of coastline came and went and soon we drove back into Croatia, only twelve miles more north. Croatia for sure had a lot more development than Montenegro, Bosnia and Albania. On the ride stopping again for pictures and a quick and nutritious meal consisting of a banana, a raw red pepper and a can of octopus.

Eventually we arrived in Split and quickly noticed the busy port area with ferries constantly going out to the resort islands such as Korcula or Hvar Islands. Immediately I went to the local tourist office to find a room to sleep and the ferry departure times to Hvar Island which was our next destination. The tourist office found us a quaint air conditioned private home with two separate bedrooms for thirty dollars each for the night. On these types of trips sleeping in private rooms is quite common for backpackers because the backpacker simply sleeps there for a short stay. That evening I ate at a restaurant having the broiled local fish (which I had no idea which fish it was), a zucchini and asparagus salad and a small gelato. The restaurant was right in the enclosed section of the city so our table was outside on the cobblestone street overlooking the huge lighted walls that at one time hundreds of years ago protected the city. Nightlife was a bit lame because Split is a port city so people come and go and I guess not really hang around to go dancing. I stopped at some local lounge to have a glass of red Croatian wine and socialize with a few of the locals, nothing really happening though. Again it was an early night because unlike Spain or Greece these countries weren't crazy party countries. In a way that was ok because it enabled us to wake up early to catch an early ferry to Hvar Island and make the most of the day.

Daily Workout

2 mile run followed by 10 sets of 10 pull-ups, 15 dips and 20 push-ups

Meals

Breakfast
Nonfat yogurt drink
Rye bread

Snack
Apple
Walnuts

Lunch
Can of octopus
Raw red pepper
Banana

Dinner
Broiled fresh fish
Zucchini and asparagus salad
Gelato

HVAR ISLAND, DALMATIAN COAST, CROATIA

Awake by eight a.m. the beautiful sunny day was started off with a three mile run along the sea overlooking the beautiful Adriatic and what a sight that is. Nothing beats that ocean breeze while going for a nice jog because the salt water breeze really opens up your lungs. The run was short but enough to wake me up and put me in a great mood thanks to that "runner's high" that I look to achieve during every workout. After the run I had breakfast which consisted of "Isopure" whey protein isolate, some fresh strawberries and a small chocolate filled croissant which was very tasty because it was hot from being freshly baked. Yes of course I know that a chocolate filled croissant is not healthy and low calorie but you have to splurge once in a while because after all we are human, right? Throughout the years I realized that you are better off cheating on your diet every once in a while to satisfy your cravings because if you don't cheat you will end up quitting your entire diet much sooner. Nowadays I cheat on my diet a little every day and I'm much happier overall because I'm not daydreaming of food all day. A little cheat here and there and you will still get in shape but without the suffering from not splurging.

That same morning we boarded our ferry on route to the famous Hvar Island, the "who's who" place in the Dalmatian coast. The ferry was pretty basic but packed with tourists and had a real good vibe to it. There were all tourists on board but we were the only Americans but that's a good thing because when you're in a foreign country you always want to see different people and especially the local people who live there. The three hour ferry ride was pleasant, it was sunny and breezy not to mention the spectacular scenery of the Adriatic Sea and its magnificent islands. Traveling especially this way is the ultimate freedom, journey and memories. When you really look at it at the end of the day all we really have are memories so the more good memories the better. Of course I was hungry again so I opted to see what the ferry's food stand had to offer. In my backpack I did have a can of octopus and an apple but I was a little tired of that food so I decided to eat something different. The food stand really didn't have anything too healthy so I ordered a hamburger without the bun and a Croatian salad which consisted of pickles and turnips. The salad was actually quite healthy. Not the best meal because hamburgers have a lot of saturated fat and calories but once in a while it is ok for a little change of pace.

As the ferry entered the dock on Hvar Island it was evident that this was a popular place because the marina was filled with yachts that came from all over the Mediterranean because each boat carried its different country flag. As soon as we boarded onto dock numerous people approached us offering rooms to sleep for the night. With a little negotiating I was able to find a place to stay right off the pier overlooking the Sea. The room didn't have air conditioning but I figured that there would be an ocean breeze all night. I ended up making a crucial mistake. Immediately following check in it was time for another "lean" meal. I ended up drinking a quart of skim milk. Skim milk has no fat and a decent amount of protein however consuming dairy products should be kept at a minimum because the lactose that's in milk quickly turns to sugar.

Next it was off to the beach. So far the sand quality of the beaches was sub par. Albanian and Montenegrin beaches were filled with small pebbles instead of sand and the beaches in Hvar Island were the same. Adriatic Sea water temperatures are probably somewhere around seventy seven degrees Fahrenheit. not bad at all but the eighty two degrees of the eastern Mediterranean Sea is a tad bit better. The main beach on Hvar Island was packed with jetsetters and stars. The sun was bright, the beach was packed and the music was right. I rented a paddle boat to not only get a little cardio but to sightsee as well. The half hour ride was nice. On the beach I just walked around from beach to beach noticing a few turning heads because having a muscular body is a rarity, especially in these type of countries. Because of my non stop and "ADD" type of personality I had to keep walking around from beach to beach and why not because there were plenty of attractive people to look at!

The beach time ended so I was off to the town market to buy some fresh vegetables, fruit, wine and low fat cheese. While shopping with the local people I noticed the many steel and wooden bars that would be perfect for my daily workout. I then asked when the fair ended so I could return later on for a workout. It turns out that it ended at eight p.m. As soon as I arrived back to my room I prepared another meal consisting of fresh low fat cheese and blackberries as my dessert. Cheese isn't the best meal but being low fat it wasn't bad because of the protein and healthy fat it had. The blackberries were a tasty carbohydrate and dessert. The meal was good enough to be a pre-workout meal because it was approaching eight p.m., the time when the fair ended so my workout could begin.

Arriving back to the fair I noticed a few stores and vendors remained open. That was fine because they would get to see a free workout! One of the stores that were open was a quaint little cheese and wine shop and everything was locally produced so I thought "hhhmmm" a nice post-workout treat! Before I began to structure my workout I looked around at the "equipment" I had to work with. Overhead steel bars would accommodate my back, biceps and abs workout while a couple of chairs would accommodate doing dips for my chest, shoulder and triceps workout. For a leg workout I would have to super set lunges with squats and calves. The workout began with super setting pull-ups with dips to push-ups to free squats to lunges to calves for ten total sets. The first five were brutal but right at the sixth set I started to feel the "runners high" kick in, exactly what I've been waiting for all along.

During the workout a small crowd of people gathered around to watch, this actually is pretty normal in these types of countries. By the ninth set I was starting to smell the cheese and wine I was about to eat, the best part of the workout. As the tenth set ended I headed straight for that wine and cheese shop and the owner was waiting outside with a glass of wine and cheese with my name written all over it. After drinking two glasses I was feeling great and that was just the beginning. A few pieces of cheese and I was set. One thing about Western Europe that I really love is the cheese and its different variety from country to country and region to region.

Some of these cheeses are years old only to refine their taste much like fine wine. Enjoying the cheese, wine and terrific company between the cheese shop owner and a few other workers. These "old school" Europeans have so much to offer as far as knowledge, the way things are and the way things used to be. I really enjoy conversing with these types of people because it's an education that no school can ever offer. Now I was feeling great because of a good workout, a few glasses of wine, some cheese, great company and most of all a nice "high" from working out. That post workout "high" is a feeling of the best euphoria without any competition! Simply put, it's unbelievable and that's what keeps me in shape for so many years consistently.

The cheese shop owner was Greek and had moved to Hvar Island years before. He was extremely friendly and after I finished my wine and cheese we all took pictures and what really made the pictures fun was the pretty female worker that I got to have my arm around. European women have that certain elegance and femininity that is very attractive. The "high" I felt from a combination between the two glasses of wine and the workout was awesome and I knew it would last for a while. Now I was jogging back to my hotel enjoying the scent of the sea breeze and the sights of the beautiful architecture of stone houses and cobblestone streets. This is seen only in old world Europe. I walked into the hostel room that we rented. Even though the room was directly in front of the sea with the window wide open it was still rather hot and without a breeze. In other words I was in for a long night. To make matters worse it turned out that directly below us was dance club. The just say that the night wouldn't be quiet. I dressed into some nice jeans, a V-neck T-shirt and a pair of flip flops. I was very comfortable. Next of course was eating a healthy meal which was fresh fruits and vegetables and a liter of water that I bought at the fair and a grilled octopus and calamari that I bought from a street vendor and of course I had told him not to use any salt because salt is what you don't want because it causes water retention. V-necks fit me well because my neck is rather large from years of wrestling so I always need that extra neck space in a shirt. That's one of the beauties of being in shape and that even the simplest clothing fits you well without any needing to camouflage any part of your body with funky clothing. Jeans, flip flops, T-shirt, slacks, suits, sweaters, etc. it all looks good on you when you're in shape.

The nightlife in Hvar Island was convenient because all of the bars and dance clubs were located next to each other right where my room was. We started off at the dance club downstairs from the room. Small but cozy and packed with tourists from all over. Surprisingly they were playing Latin music and that was perfect for me because for the past year I had been taking "Bachata", "Merengue" and "Salsa" Latin dance lessons. Eventually I knew the dance classes would come in handy and where better a place than on Hvar Island? It was evident that there were no Latin dancers in the dance club and that made it even better for me because I definitely was no "Fred Estair" on the dance floor. The fact that the place was filled with people who had no idea how to dance Latin now made me look like an expert and this I am not even close to because I almost have two left feet.

While drinking my vodka and club soda I noticed in the far corner of the dance floor I noticed an attractive woman that I needed to approach. She spoke no English but she did speak French and I was fluent in French so the first move I was taking her to the dance floor. She knew nothing about Latin dance and I knew only the basics but that was enough to properly lead her though all of the spins of Salsa dancing. Nevertheless she really loved it and was smiling the entire time. One thing I can guarantee to anyone is that with me they will have a lot of fun because I am that type of person, always upbeat and adventurous. We had a great time dancing a few songs. Definitely a great day followed by an even a better night. Before going to sleep I walked along the beach that was packed with all night party goers. Going to sleep was impossible because the club directly below my room was stilled packed and the music was still blasting. Finally the noise of the music and people singing outside ended at around five in the morning. Even though it was now quiet I still couldn't sleep because the room was too hot. The next day I knew would be difficult on two hours sleep. Rest is so important because without sufficient rest the following day you are like a "zombie" so you end up losing out on so much that day plus you're not in a great mood either. That morning at about nine in the morning I began my three mile run along the coast so I could admire the sea and the gorgeous yachts that came from all over the Mediterranean. In a few hours we would be leaving on the ferry back to Split, Croatia.

HVAR ISLAND, CROATIA

Meals

Breakfast
Hamburger (no bun)
Croatian salad with beets and radishes

Lunch
Liter of skim milk

Snack
Low fat cheese
Blackberries

Dinner
Cured cheese
Red wine

Evening snack
Grilled octopus and calamari

Raw cucumber
Banana

Nightlife
Vodka with club soda

Exercise

Complete Body Exercise
Super Set
10 Sets pull-ups, dips, Indian pushups and squats
3 Mile morning run

Leaving the island and heading to Split was a lot easier than leaving the paradise of Budva Beach. On the ferry I had a liter of water, a can of sardines and an apple. Yes it does sound like a strange meal but it is complete and will compliment your physique. Sardines may have a strong odor but they are packed with healthy Omega-3 fats. Whenever on a trip it's very important to eat healthy fats, fiber and protein. Eating like this will not only keep you lean but light as well thanks to the vegetables. Never will you feel that sluggishness you get after eating that huge and unhealthy meal that your average person eats. Don't forget that your physique either makes the vacation practically excellent. Definitely it seems as though you get more out of your vacation when you are in shape. As an example, years ago when I was twenty two years old I was involved in a really bad motorcycle accident. The injuries that I sustained included broken bones, numerous lacerations, broken sternum, collapsed lung, damaged liver and internal bleeding. It was critical and the doctors said that I would've been dead if I wasn't so physically strong. The day of the accident I weighed a fairly lean 205 pounds and after an extended stay in the hospital I ended up being discharged and the day that I left my weight was down to a soft and flabby 168 pounds! The minute that I looked in the mirror I was disgusted by seeing how I lost my entire physique!

Nevertheless it took me about six months of working out and dieting to get my body back into shape but first let me tell you how I had felt being out of shape, soft and flabby. I was discharged on June 28th an immediately after my release everyone kept asking what had happened because they barely recognized me. A month later I left for Spain to visit my friends and family and of course they were shocked at what they saw also. Going to the beach then to the nightlife was a daily ritual and for the first time I wasn't in shape at all and it felt terrible! My quality of life was way worse being out of shape and as if I was missing out on so much more. Not a good feeling at all. Regardless and against the doctors wishes I began to exercise and eat right daily. As the months went by I was feeling better and better every day. Then finally after six months I was "me" again. Feeling positive and energetic once again. Now the quality of life had finally returned. From the span of six months life changed to the better dramatically.

From that point on I vowed to myself to always stay in shape. Now it was different from my original reason to be in shape; to do well in sports, look cool and impress the women. My new reasons for being in shape now were all about energy, positive attitude, feeling lighter and most of all to improve the quality of life. After this breakthrough it was now much easier to get into shape and maintain it all throughout. So now we can begin thinking about quality of life.

SPLIT, CROATIA

Upon arriving at the boat terminal in Split I walked over to a fruit stand to eat grapes with a can of salmon that I had bought in Hvar Island. After eating that nutritious meal we began walking though the old town which was surrounded by fifty feet walls. Taking many pictures and walking around just absorbing the culture.

That day I took the day off of training because every now and then it's beneficial to take a day off. The "old city" was beautiful with its thousand year history. After a few hours of walking and buying souvenirs it was time for another meal. This time I would eat two cups of non-fat, plain and sugar-free Greek yogurt. Greek yogurt has more protein and fewer carbohydrates than conventional yogurt thus making it a better choice for your body.

Next was a taxi ride to Split Airport where we then parted ways. Eric was heading back to the U.S. and I was headed to Spain, starting with a night in Barcelona. After saying goodbye we both parted ways. It was definitely a great trip and Eric is a great person to travel with because he is neat, organized, easy going and keeps in shape also. In other words we have a lot in common.

Purchasing a one way ticket to Barcelona was fast and easy but before I boarded the plane I had to eat something healthy. Right next to me in the airport was a cafeteria. There I ordered a salad that had a hard boiled egg and tuna. Of course I didn't eat the yolk which made it to be another lean meal hence another day of being in shape and unique!

The three hour flight went quickly and I didn't eat the terrible airplane food which consisted of a piece of ham and cheese and buttered bread. Nothing could be worse for your body. Landing in Barcelona was pleasant because of the weather and the fact that this would be my first time in this magnificent city. As soon as I was off the plane I boarded a taxi and gave him the directions of a hostel in the center of town. Now in the fifty dollar hostel I telephoned Jennifer who was a friend of a college wrestling buddy of mine and his name was Russ Terlicki who happens to be a terrific promoter in Manhattan. Russ is always in the limelight and knows everyone. Never meeting Jennifer before had no bearing because I can get along with everyone, I'm really a people's person.

As soon as Jennifer arrived we were off to the port side right on the Mediterranean where all of the clubs happen to be. Sure enough the place was jumping. There were several dance clubs that were next to each other and they were all top of the line. Nothing compares to Spain's nightlife! Especially anywhere in Europe. Spain's nightlife never stops. It usually begins a two a.m. and ends by eight a.m.! Spain has the perfect combination of beautiful style, fantastic food and a lot of "Fiesta" which means "party" in Spanish. While in the club before ordering a "Bacardi" 151 with diet soda I asked for a water to mix some whey protein powder that I had in my pocket wrapped in plastic. The music was great and Jennifer turned out to be really cool. Nevertheless we had a great time!

SPLIT, CROATIA MEAL ITINERARY

Meals

Breakfast
Canned sardines
Apple

Snack
Canned salmon
Grapes

Lunch
2 Cups of non fat, sugar-free Greek yogurt

Dinner
Salad with hard boiled egg and tuna

BARCELONA, SPAIN

Late night snack
Whey protein isolate with water

Nightlife
"Bacardi rum 151" mixed with diet soda

Exercise (at a local gym)

Legs
Superset
4 Sets leg extension 15 reps
4 Sets hamstring leg curls 15 reps
4 Sets walking lunges 10 steps
Superset
4 Sets smith machine squats 8 reps
4 Sets standing leg curl 8 reps
4 sets donkey calf raises 20 reps

As the early riser that I am the first thing I did was have breakfast. The hostel had a small breakfast but I managed to eat six hard boiled egg whites and two pieces of toast. Water and coffee is usually what I drink every morning. After breakfast and before I were to check out I was off to walking the streets of Barcelona to find a gym and sightsee at the same time. The streets were absolutely beautiful with the gorgeous monuments, architecture and trees. The climate was perfect. Barcelona must be among the best places to live all over the world! Sure enough there was a gym right in front of me. The daily training fee was very high at around twenty-five Euros. Regardless the facility was nice and the personal trainer there quickly started a conversation with me which was fine because he was very polite and I enjoy talking to new people. This is common because in most countries there are very few people that are in that type of shape. Most of the time they ask you questions about your diet and exercise regimen. This personal trainer noticed my cauliflower ear and black eye from an MMA fight almost two weeks earlier. He happened to be a fan of mixed martial arts. We had an extensive conversation which we both enjoyed. Making friends while traveling can be interesting because not only do you make new contacts but sometimes you can hit it off great right from the beginning and feel very comfortable talking about things you wouldn't normally talk about with your friends from home.

The workout ended then the conversation did and after showering at the gym I would walk around to go sightseeing. A nice workout and a great "runner's high" equals a fun walk sightseeing around the metropolis of Barcelona. The streets were amazing and the street life was second to none. Europe in general and especially Spain has unbelievable street life. No matter which part of town you're in you will always see well dressed people socializing and having fun in cafés, restaurants and bars. People there really know how to live. For me the best part of Barcelona was along the beach. Buildings, restaurants, night clubs, shops and people are all around that beachfront area making it absolutely spectacular! It was now approaching two p.m. and it was time for another meal. It was close to lunch time so I began looking for a café that seemed fairly healthy. At first walking into this little "Mom and Pop" café I noticed all of the exotic "Iberian" ham hanging from the ceiling with strings. Not the healthiest food but I decided to order a "pincho" of the Iberian ham which Spaniards call "Jamon Iberico". Ordering only a tiny sized "pincho" was the smallest portion, sort of like a mini appetizer if not even less. Along with the ham I also ordered a glass of white wine, bottled water, "café con leche", an anchovy and tuna salad with hearts of palm and a garlic soup. A very tasty meal and even healthy enough to keep my body in shape and energized because I love "maximizing" my vacations.

Immediately following the "cultural" meal I needed to head out to the airport to catch a flight to Spain's west coast city Vigo. At the airport of course I purchased the least expensive ticket with some generic brand airline called Spanair. Once arriving to the gate for departure I noticed a long line because with this airline you aren't assigned a seat, seating is on a "first come first serve" basis, certainly not to my liking. Once on the plane it was time to eat again and this time it would be fresh asparagus that I purchased from a street vegetable cart and a can of squid that I purchased at the airport grocery store. With a liter of water the meal was tasty, efficient and completely healthy. It's very important to eat healthy while traveling especially to avoid sicknesses you can get from unhealthy foods. The people on the plane looked at me like I was crazy because of the odd meal that I was eating. This happens to me often but they usually point at the muscle in my arm and then at my food which means to them that I eat like this in order to build and maintain a healthy body.

Landing in Vigo was beautiful due to the mountains and views of the Atlantic Ocean. Vigo is located in "Galicia" which is the northwestern region of Spain, adjacent to Portugal and the Atlantic Ocean. Then while taking the taxi to our house in "Playa de Areas" I kept admiring the gorgeous views of "Las Rias Baixas" which are the tremendous bays that connect into the Atlantic Ocean. As soon as the taxi dropped me off I changed into my workout clothes and headed straight for the gym that I had built in our house. Chest, back and shoulders would be the workout followed by relaxing in the Jacuzzi then a shower. Meal time again but this time I wanted a change from the usual "backpacking" quick and efficient meals. Finally I was in the comfort of a home so I made a shake consisting whey protein, almonds, grapes and a little bit of oats. Blended with ice and to me it tastes just as good as a milkshake! For me blended home made protein shakes are a huge treat.

By now I had called my friend Marcos and he was headed over to visit me. I have several friends there but I can only call one at a time or else they all come at once and stay for hours on end eating and celebrating. Their diets are tasty but not conducive for having a "six-pack". Marcos, his brother in law "Sergio" and myself got on my bicycles and headed for town for some "tapas" a few kilometers away. My friends have to pay the price whenever they come to visit because I always make them exercise, in this case it was a bicycle ride. They may complain a bit but once I squeeze their arms and shake my head side to side meaning "not acceptable" in other words they must get into some type of shape. They laugh but agree. In my home there is a policy and that is that all my guests must exercise (my 96 year old grandmother is excluded) with me and eat healthy as well. Hopefully I can start a trend!

My friends and I always have fun because when health and exercise is involved everything happens to be more productive and entertaining. Fun is my middle name and let's just say that I might have had a little too much fun in my life! Sure enough when friends stop buy we play handball, soccer, basketball, boxing, bicycling or weight training. Right after exercising I make sure to feed them something healthy such as a protein shake. Believe it or not they not only have fun but several of them begin to exercise regular with me. Often I am looked at as a little crazy due to my disciplined regiment but once I show them my way of life so they can experience it themselves then all of a sudden they are on board with my program. Not only do I truly believe in my methods of diet and nutrition but people are convinced rather easily because they see me physically fit and mentally energized and sharp.

Not to get too far off our ride we bicycled into the port side town of Portonovo. A small, quaint fishermen village that it is makes for fresh fish and seafood that is readily available in the small family owned businesses that are right in front of the Atlantic Ocean. We entered a small little tavern and ordered a few "tapas" which are portions of food that are smaller portions than appetizers but larger than "pinchos". The specials that were fresh caught that day that we ordered were "chocos" which are squid, we also ordered "navajas" which are "razor clams" and finally we asked for a "tapa" of "gambas a la plancha" which are grilled jumbo shrimp. When ordering I always specify "no salt" because the extra sodium causes water retention which makes you look "bloated" and "puffy". Also we ordered "Albarino" wine which is a locally made white wine. Spaniards always stress the importance of drinking white wine with fish and seafood and red wine with meat because it improves digestion and kills the bacteria that is in the fish, seafood and meat. There you have it! A great tasting cultural meal that is very healthy, high in protein and Omega-3 fats. A "win win situation" for the three of us!

Let's face it that big part of life and vacation is eating the different foods that are offered everywhere. This is how my methods of getting into shape differ than most others because I stress enjoyment and culture which includes doing the exercises and eating the foods that you enjoy. Most other personal trainers instruct their clients to do such things as I wouldn't such as eating the same foods all of the time and without being the clients choice of foods and having their clients use a treadmill or stationary bicycle as their only options to do cardio. Basically the way I differ from other trainers is simple in that most trainers instruct their clients on what to eat and how to exercise giving them no choices what so ever. On the other hand I treat all of my clients on a case by case basis by spending a lot of time working with their needs, goals and preference of food choices and exercise options. Constructing a complete itinerary for getting into shape that is custom fitted to their lifestyles.

Now back to our eating "tapas" and drinking wine in that we had nutritious meals but most of all we enjoyed ourselves without feeling deprived of tasty foods. Another advantage of taking bicycles when going out to eat is you get to burn off the calories during the ride back home. Biking the way home we stopped at a popular lounge in the next beach front town called "Sanxenxo". The place was packed with people so it didn't need much convincing to have a drink and socialize. Even on a Sunday night you will always find nightlife. Spain's nightlife has a worldwide reputation as among the best. Parties and festivals and food are a part of Spain's culture. At the lounge ordered an "aguardiente" with ice. "Aguardiente" is the alcohol that is made from the left over grape skins from the wine making process. I made sure that my friends ordered reduced calorie cocktails as well. The night was over and what a productive first day at our vacation home that was!

Home Gym Workout, Playa de Areas

Chest
5 Sets incline dumbbell press 12 reps
5 Sets pec-deck 12 reps

Shoulders
5 Sets dumbbell lateral raises 15 reps
5 Sets front military press 10 reps

Back
5 Sets bent over rows 10 reps
5 Sets wide-grip pull-ups 12 reps

Meals

Breakfast
6 Hard boiled egg whites
2 Pieces of toast
Coffee

Lunch
Iberian ham
Salad with anchovies, tuna and hearts of palm
Glass of wine

Snack
Can of squid
Asparagus

Snack
Shake with whey protein isolate, almonds, grapes, and oats

Dinner
Navajas (razor clams)
Grilled jumbo shrimp
Squid
White wine

Café con leche desnatada (espresso with frothed skim milk)

Nightlife
Aguardiente on the rocks

PLAYA DE AREAS, SANXENXO, SPAIN

Monday morning I was awake by eight in the morning, at about the same time that it becomes light out. I know what you thinking because eight a.m. is kind of late for day break but where Galicia lies on the map calls for later days. In June and July it becomes dark at eleven p.m.! People usually go to the beach at five p.m. and stay until nine p.m. Simply said it's just a "later" lifestyle in general. My usual morning starts with an espresso coffee followed by a six mile bike ride to go grocery shopping at the "plaza" which is the open market. As soon as I get home I prepare breakfast which today was egg whites and oatmeal. This day being my first morning at the vacation home I had a lot of work cut out for me with setting everything up for the summer such as the gym, Jacuzzi, lawn mower, boat, quad, motocross bike and motorcycle. When these items sit around unattended from one season to the next they become damaged, especially the engines from not being started in a while.

My good friend Marcos came by and our first project was fixing and starting my Polaris quad. We charged the battery and changed the oil and spark plug and sure enough it started! I drove it out from the garage to let the motor run for a while. Like a fool I didn't leave the parking brake on and while walking into the garage I heard the quad rolling down our driveway! A very steep fifty yard hill! The quad zipped down but luckily crashed into one of the granite pillars in front of the house. Another five inches to the right and the quad would have crashed into the neighbor's house! Now imagine a five hundred pound quad at about thirty miles per hour going straight down the hill with no driver? Not a pretty site. It turns out that for a thousand dollars everything was fixed, the quad and the pillar. Definitely embarrassing!

After the quad we went to start the motocross bike, a Yamaha YZ 250. being that the YZ was a two-stroke and had no battery it started right up after a few kicks after changing the spark plug. "Two down and two to go" so next vehicle to start was the Kawasaki ZX11 motorcycle. We needed to clean the four spark plugs, change the oil, bleed the brakes and charge the battery. An hour later it started right up and I was excited because I love speeding and riding wheelies with the ZX. It was time for another meal and that would be farmed Checkmate"speed boat and the motor was an outboard Mercury EFI 2.5 which is a racing two-stroke with 280 horsepower. The boat is good for seventy miles per hour which is fast for a boat. We charged up the two batteries and cleaned the six spark plugs. After a few cranks it started too. Now I needed to have the quad tow it to the boat launch ramp in order to be stored at the marina. Even though the quad was damaged it could still do the job of towing the boat. After coming back home it was meal-time, a boiled octopus we ate that Marcos caught and a lettuce, olive and goat cheese salad.

Where I live there in Spain we are on the Atlantic coastline next to many small "fisherman" villages. The area is a dream come true with the beautiful green mountains, pristine shoreline, "fisherman" villages, farms and the many wine vineyards. Now it would be time to exercise and a few people stopped by to join us. When I'm in town the word gets out and people start coming over to visit and workout. Actually when they visit I make them exercise! They usually only raised chicken breast with onions and broccoli. Marcos and I ate a great meal and right after we were ready to start the boat. Eating small meals never slows you down after a meal because the food is light hence you wont feel sluggish. The boat was a complain for the first fifteen minutes. We all had a good biceps, triceps and calf workout. Following the workout we had whey protein shakes with fruit and oatmeal. The rest of the day I worked around the house preparing for the vacation.

That evening we went to dinner at a restaurant. In Spain dinner is at midnight believe it or not. Quickly you become accustomed to the later schedule that the Spaniards have. At the restaurant I had a salad with prawns and "rape a la plancha" which is grilled Monkfish. Always a glass of white wine with the seafood. After dinner I rode my motorcycle into town for the nightlife. Every night in the summer is a good night to go out. The "muelle" which means pier is always packed with partygoers and of course it's not hard to twist my arm to go out! The "muelle" has ten or twelve clubs and lounges and all of them are packed with a different crowd. Some of the clubs have long lines to get in but that's never a problem for me because I usually offer the bouncer a free membership at my gym or ask if they need to spar with me in the boxing ring or wrestling mat. They usually appreciate the gesture but rarely follow up, especially the sparring part. Nevertheless my offerings usually get me the red carpet treatment for the rest of the summer. A few of my friends own clubs there which is another plus but the only drawback is they always ask them to tell their customers my stories of something crazy in my life such as a few high speed police chases on my motorcycle or some of travel to remote country stories, especially when there was some type of danger or "brushes with the law" that were often experienced. People tend to get a kick out of these types of stories. I must admit telling them isn't as much fun as living them especially when the story had a safe ending.

The night was going well especially after drinking a Bacardi 151 with diet soda. After the nightlife everyone either goes home at four a.m. or to another club. Usually I go home and end up driving a stranger home because people there often ask you for a ride home especially when you have a fast and sleek motorcycle. I never have a problem driving anyone home as long as A) it's not a guy and B) not an overweight women because I'm worried about her plastering into me if I have to slam on the brakes or even worse is that I like riding wheelies but with a heavy person on back the motorcycle is likely to flip over backward. Plus if they are overweight perhaps they should consider walking back in order to burn calories.

So this leads me to who qualifies to get a ride home and that is attractive women of course! For a treat I like scaring them and riding a few wheelies while riding them home. Women usually scream at first but after you slow down and drop them off they already miss the excitement of danger! Contrary to what they say, women much rather a fearless, exciting thrill seeker rather than your average guy who is afraid to take risks in life.

Daily Exercise Routine

Biceps
4 Sets dumbbell hammer curls 12 reps
4 Sets dumbbell preacher curls 12 reps
4 Sets straight bar curls 12 reps

Triceps
4 Sets lying triceps extension 12 reps
4 Sets triceps pushdown 12 reps
4 Sets kickbacks 12 reps

Abs
Roman chair leg raises 50 reps

Meals

Breakfast
½ cup of Liquid egg whites
2/3 cup of "Old-fashioned" oatmeal
Espresso coffee with skim milk

Lunch
6 oz. Broiled Chicken breast
Sautéed (in water) broccoli and onions

Snack
Pulpo a la Gallega (boiled octopus served in olive oil and paprika)
Salad with lettuce, tomato, cucumber, olives and goat cheese with olive oil and white balsamic vinegar

Dinner
Rape a la plancha (grilled monkfish with fresh lemon)
Salad with steamed prawns

Nightlife
Bacardi 151 with diet soda

PLAYA DE AREAS, SPAIN

As any other morning I am up by eight a.m. and eager to take on the day. After a café con leche desnatada I decided on going for a morning kayak ride to switch up my cardio. The beach there has several kayaks on the sand. These kayaks are owned by the local town people whether for recreation, sport or fishing but it's ok to simply borrow one as long as it's used responsibly meaning no damage. A forty five minute kayak ride to the "mejioneras" (these wooden floats that are used to harvest mussels). The "mejioneras" are usually a few hundred meters from the shore. Definitely a good back workout too. By the time the ride finished I was starving because cardio is best done in the early morning on an empty stomach. At home I then prepared high fiber pancakes and egg whites. The high fiber pancakes are a real treat and they qualify as a "healthy meal". After breakfast I called a few friends to invite them to go waterskiing now that my boat was already in the water at the local marina. Sure enough a few said yes. Now it was time to prepare the meals for the long day out on the ocean. Keeping it simple I just brought two cans of tuna, two raw peppers, grapes and a few liters of water. As soon as I arrived to my boat it was time for another meal so quickly I ate the tuna, raw pepper and a few grapes.

The day on the boat now began. We drove across the "Ria" (bay) where the water was calmer. Driving a boat at seventy miles per hour is so much fun! We found a calm place and began taking turns water skiing. Once it was my turn I was a bit nervous because it's been a year since I last water-skied. It went well though as I mono skied as well. Of course we were hungry so I drove the boat into a quaint little fisherman village and ordered "necoras" which are boiled crabs, "vieras" which are scallops and "salpicon" which is a steamed seafood salad with hard-boiled eggs. Very unique and tasty meal but most of all it was lean. Riding home fast as the sun goes down is an experience in itself. We docked then I rode my bicycle home to meet my friends so we can eat and train. We exercised on the speed and heavy bags for thirty minutes then we started training back and biceps with a few sets of forearms at the end. The workout was nice and having cool music in the background with a beautiful view of the Atlantic Ocean only added to the experience. The workout ended and the "runner's high" began, the best part of training! As for our post workout meal we decided to have protein shakes with walnuts, banana, oatmeal and whey protein isolate. A workout completed followed by a lean shake I was ready to prepare for the night of fun. That night we decided on getting a little drunk so the perfect idea was walking to the beach and having a "queimada". To prepare a "queimada" we would need a very large clay pot, "aguardiente" (grain alcohol), lemons, apples, oranges, coffee beans and brown sugar. This sounds like something strange but it's a ritual in Spain and the process of making it is what makes the evening. The process begins with laying the pot on the beach and filling it with slices apples, oranges, lemons, coffee beans and "aguardiente". As soon as the contents are added you then use a match to light it on fire. As it's burning slowly stir and occasionally sip it to see if it is still to strong for your taste. As the alcohol burns it begins to taste less potent which is then you add sugar to burn in the flame. The sugar will burn hence caramelizing on top of the contents. Everyone around the fire uses a cup to dip in and drink. Everyone slowly but surely gets a little drunk as they drink, talk and watch the fire. It turns out to be a great night which is exactly what we did. Stirring and drinking the flaming drink while admiring the ocean at night. Once again it was a beautiful night of culture and memories. What a fantastic vacation so far!

QUIMADA EVENING

Meals

Breakfast
Coffee with skim milk
Cup of egg whites
High fiber pancakes

Snack
Can of light tuna in water
Raw red pepper
Grapes

Lunch
Can of light tuna in water
Raw red pepper
Grapes

Snack
Steamed crab
Lemon broiled scallops
Seafood salad with hard-boiled egg

Dinner (post workout meal)
Protein shake made with whey protein isolate, walnuts, oats,
banana, ice, water

Exercise

Morning kayak ride 45 minutes
Evening exercise routine
Speed bag 15 minutes
Heavy bag 15 minutes

Back
5 Sets T-bar rows 15 reps
5 Sets dead-lifts 8 reps
5 Sets dumbbell rows 10 reps
5 Sets lat machine pull-downs 10 reps

Biceps
4 Sets preacher curls 15 reps
4 Sets cable curls 12 reps
4 Sets hammer curls 10 reps

Forearms
5 Sets forearm curls 20 reps

Nightlife
Queimada (aguardiente" (grape skin alcohol), coffee beans,
fruit, sugar

ISLAS CIES
Definitely a cultural evening due to the "queimada" and once again no
hangover because I always drink a lot of water whenever I drink alcohol

and that is the secret. Waking up in the morning with the fresh smell of the Atlantic is a pleasure that words can't describe. The views where I live are like what you see on postcards, breath taking! This morning I chose to go on a forty minute run through the mountains that are located behind our house. These mountains are great for running because they overlook the Atlantic Ocean which provide for great scenery and the mountains are filled with eucalyptus trees which provide for an invigorating scent that helps your breathing and clears your sinuses. "Vick's" vapor rub is made from eucalyptus so you could imagine how good it feels jogging through that scent. The run ended and I felt great.

Not enough could be said about how beneficial it is to run in the early morning. The "runner's high" you get will last you for hours, a pleasant tingling feeling throughout your body. Breakfast was two soft boiled eggs, an apricot and two pieces of rye bread along with coffee. As soon as I finished breakfast I needed to prepare for our day trip to "Islas Cies". These islands are gorgeous let alone the main beach on the island was rated one of the top ten beaches in the world! That enough should tell you about the islands. The ride to the island would take about an hour to get there by boat therefore we needed to pack enough food to last us an entire day. Bringing a spear gun would be a good idea in order to catch either a fish or octopus which are abound around this island. It would be a great idea to eat freshly caught fish or seafood as our main afternoon meal. Years ago when I was thirteen, fourteen and fifteen years old I went fishing nearly everyday both by using a fishing line or spear gun. As a kid fishing on my motorboat was a lot of fun but then later on after buying my first speedboat all that changed because now I was waterskiing and speeding around instead of fishing. Nevertheless I am scuba certified but I would rather fish without the oxygen tanks and use my own lungs for oxygen in order to get into better physical shape. Before we headed out on the long journey it was time to eat again. We kept it simple and ate turkey breast, squash and blackberries for dessert. Turkey is always a wise option to eat because it is extremely low in fat and high in protein. Another plus to eating turkey breast especially at night because it has the amino acid trypto-phan which relaxes you.

We then bicycled two to the small little fishermen village called "Raxo" where my boat is anchored. Bicycling there is quite a challenge because of all of the steep hills. The benefit of bicycling on steep hills is that it provides "interval" cardio training meaning "easy, hard, easy, hard" and at never the same heart rate. Starting up and heading out is always the fun because the views from a boat are spectacular. Leaving the "Ria de Pontevedra" and heading into the open Atlantic Ocean is not easy because of the Atlantic's immense waves. The waves were fun only because they were a bit dangerous. Driving the boat south through the Atlantic after leaving the "Ria de Pontevedra" we passed the "Ria de Aldan" which is small and quaint which I love and to make it even bet-ter are the hidden empty beaches and caves that are right on the water that you can enter with your boat to see and listen to the bats that live in the caves. After the "Ria de Aldan" we next passed on our left hand side was another "Ria" called the "Ria de Vigo" which is much larger. Vigo is the largest city in the area with around five hundred thou-sand people. Vigo has a large shipping port where I have sent shipping containers to from the U.S. Vigo also has the airport where I usual-ly fly into. The city is very near the border with Portugal. Forty five minutes had passed since we began the journey and soon enough we saw the gorgeous islands on our right hand side. "Cies Islands" were loaded with white sandy beaches, trees and huge rocks which make it all in all spectacular! We dropped the anchor very near the shore so we could hop off the boat and walk waist deep to the shore. Setting up a few towels and a radio I grabbed the spear gun to go fishing. The under water scenery was pristine with fish abound. Quickly I caught a medium sized Bass fish followed by a Whiting fish and finally my favorite catch of all which is octopus. We dug a small hole in the sand and filled it with tree branches with a metal grate on top to make the BBQ. Cooking freshly caught fish was just as fun as eating it. Fish and seafood are loaded with protein and healthy Omegs-3 fats. Eating the

fish and octopus with a glass of white wine and some pears for dessert that we picked off a tree on the island made the entire
trip well worth it!

The ride home went quicker because there were less waves being that it was later in the day. Docking the boat in "Raxo" was the easy part compared to the bicycle ride home. Once arriving home I prepared a good pre-workout protein shake which consisted of whey protein isolate, peanut butter, oats, figs, ice and water. A light shake forty five minutes before resistance exercise provides constant energy that will last the entire workout. Training chest, triceps, and abs would be finished in thirty minutes because we would superset the exercises. Surely thirty minutes flew by and now I felt re-energized. Our post-exercise meal was "Tortilla Espanola" which means "Spanish omelet. Of course changes to the recipe would be necessary in order for it to be a healthy meal so the egg yolks were exchanged for egg whites and the white potatoes were exchanged for sweet potatoes and squash. Adding squash is a fantastic way to add fiber and satiety to your meal because eating vegetables really has no drawbacks what so ever. A few figs for dessert finished the meal. It was already late and I was exhausted from a complete day of excitement and adventure so staying home, skipping the nightlife and going to sleep was the best option. Overall it was a fantastic day with memories that will last me a lifetime.

"ISLAS CIES"

Meals

8 A.M. Early morning coffee
Breakfast
2 Soft-boiled eggs
2 Slices of rye bread
Apricots
Coffee

Snack
Plain fried turkey breast
Squash
Blackberries

Lunch
BBQ Whiting fish
BBQ Striped bass fish
BBQ Octopus
Pears
White wine

Snack (pre-exercise)
Shake blended with whey protein isolate, peanut butter, oats, figs, ice, and water

Dinner (post-exercise)
Spanish omelet made with egg whites, sweet potato and butternut squash
Figs

Exercise

Chest
Super set all three chest exercises
5 Sets of incline dumbbell flies 20 reps
5 Sets of push-ups 20 reps
5 Sets of dips 20 reps

Triceps
Super set both exercises
5 Sets of seated triceps extension 20 reps

5 Sets of diamond push-ups 20 reps

Abs
Leg raises 75 reps

Cardio
Morning mountain run 40 minutes
Afternoon bicycle ride 4 miles

ISLA DE ONS

Not going out to the clubs last night was a good idea. Not seeing attractive well dressed women was the downside of staying in last night but having a good night sleep is worth "a thousand words". After a good night sleep your day is so much more productive and your mood is better as well. Drinking no alcohol makes for much deeper "REM" sleep which is deeper sleep. Feeling like a million bucks at eight in the morning means that you are off to a great start. Filled with energy I decided to take the mountain bike on a nice forty minute steep mountain ride. The fresh pine and eucalyptus trees provided the fresh scent that would last the entire ride. By doing different types of cardio each time your body constantly remains in a state of shock which is the object because shocking your system causes the most physical improvement.

The mountain bike ride ended and I couldn't wait to get back home to make a shake for breakfast. Soon after I had to take my bicycle into town to go shopping. Food shopping in Spain is way different than food shopping in the U.S. because the food labels are entirely different. Buying the basic chicken breast, eggs, and wheat bran is pretty easy. Once you want to be specific and buy non-fat feta cheese, unprocessed wheat bran, high fiber, low calorie wraps and sweet potatoes you will have en extremely difficult time finding these items if even finding them at all. Whenever abroad you must improvise with your diet and training in order to be in shape. Food shopping in the "plaza" is quite an experience because it's an outdoor market loaded with fresh fish, meat, cheese, vegetables and fruit. The vendors are still dressed in either their fishing outfits or farming clothes. The vendors are all local people so everyone is on a first name basis and they always call me "el Americano" which means "the American". I bought food for the day which included vegetables, "navajas" which are razor clams, mussels and turkey breast.

Following breakfast consisting of egg whites, high fiber cereal and cured lamb cheese we prepared more meals for another long day out on the boat to the island of "Ons". "Isla de Ons" is primarily known for its octopus that is caught right on its shores. At home I boiled the mussels and razor clams and packed a few liters of drinking water. "Isla de Ons" is not too far away and you can see the island right from our balcony and it's about a half hour away on boat. "Cies" and "Ons" are islands on the Atlantic that are now considered national reserve parks. Driving to the island is always fun because speed is my passion and jumping over the waves only adds to the adventure. As soon as we docked it was a nice feeling to be on a remote island in the Atlantic. It was already lunch time so we headed to the local restaurant which was only a short walk away. We ordered the fresh octopus of the day along with monk fish and salad. To drink we had what goes best with fish and seafood which is white wine. Once we ordered the food I did my usual and walked into the kitchen to ask the cook not to use any salt or grease in any of the food. The chef was a nice "old school" woman who got a chuckle out of me walking into the kitchen. She immediately understood that I was into health and fitness once she grabbed my arm. It seems that the "old timers" get a kick out of squeezing your muscle because they think it was attributed from working construction. To maintain your health it is important to always ask for your food to be prepared plain or with lemon but never salt or too many spices.

The food was great as was the experience and right after we walked around the island noticing all of the tourists and backpackers enjoying themselves drinking and some of them were smoking hashish which is quite common in Spain. I was never into any type of smoking because of my athletic lifestyle.

The ride home was a blast because the water was calmer so I could push the boat to seventy miles per hour which feels a lot faster on the water. Before stopping home we made a stop at "Combarro" beach to have a coffee at a café that must have been four hundred years old and on a rock right over the water. Once at home it was exercise time and followed by a few rounds of sparring and hitting the heavy bag. When training finished I ate the seafood that I had boiled earlier along with oatmeal. Getting ready for the nightlife felt great because the "runner's high" from training was still fresh. The pier had a nice crowd both classy and well dressed. Drinking two "Kalimochas" which is red wine mixed with diet soda was enough to get me going and the fun would begin. A nice evening but I was stuck driving home a woman that was hitchhiking which is quite normal in Spain. To scare her of course I had to pop a few wheelies which definitely did the trick. She loved it though!

"ISLA DE ONS"

Meals

Breakfast
Shake with whey protein isolate, almonds, oats, banana, ice and water
Coffee

Lunch
Octopus in vinaigrette dressing
Monk fish grilled in lemon
Salad with olives, lamb cheese, olive oil, lettuce and tomato

Snack
Steamed mussels
Razor clams
Goat cheese
Corn on the cob

Post-workout meal
Steamed seafood
Oatmeal

Nightlife
2 "Kalimochas" which is red wine mixed with diet soda

Exercise

Early morning bicycle ride 5 miles
Evening sparring 5 rounds and 5 rounds of heavy bag

Legs
5 Sets lunges 10 steps
5 Sets hack squats 12 reps
5 Sets hamstring curls 15 reps
5 Sets seated calf raises 20 reps

Neck
Lying neck lifts 100 reps

FIESTAS DEL ALBARINO

Strolling in at four in the morning is actually considered early for Spain's standards of nightlife. Just to give you an idea of how Spaniards live for starters dinner is at around midnight. After dinner the people start off there evenings in a few different bars at around two a.m. then at about four-thirty a.m. the crowd moves on to the nightclubs until around seven-thirty a.m. Crazy isn't it! However the early riser that I am when I go to the local coffee shop at around eight-thirty a.m. I usually see a lot of club goers stopping for a coffee on there way home. Then between ten a.m. and noon the streets are empty because everyone is still sleeping as with there siesta they take during the mid-afternoon. All in all their life is very unique to say the least.

Waking up early again and with not much sleep I had breakfast and coffee because soon after a few friends were coming over to wrestle and spar. My friends Marcos, Gabby and Pablo stopped by for a late-morning workout. We warmed up with a few rounds of jump rope followed by wrestling and finally some light Muay Thai sparring. A lot of fun especially when it was over we picked a few apples and figs from our garden to put in the shake. Fresh fruit is delicious. Today there would be no boat ride which worked out fine especially because the gasoline is more than six dollars a gallon! Instead I took a nice bike ride to a far away beach where I could sit down in some small family owned tavern and order fresh oysters, squid and prawns. Of course I had asked the waiter to grill everything without oil or salt. With a glass of white wine and a side order of "pimientos de Padron" which are fried hot locally grown peppers but the waiter kindly asked the cook to grill them instead. Grilling but never frying.

On the long ride home I stopped for a sugar-free ice cream with whipped cream. I know that it's not the healthiest but you do have to live it up a little. It was now time for a resistance workout and the children's park right on the beach was the perfect place. My usual push-pull body weight workout was completed in a half hour and it did reinvigorate me. Later at home I ate salmon with whole grain pasta then prepared for the evening. I was now headed to the "fiestas del albarino" for a night of fun with my friends. This event consisted of many booths and in each booth was a farmer who is giving away cups of his home grown wine. I had to take my motorcycle their because the streets were packed with people but they would all move aside as I passed with my motorcycle. Going from booth to booth was the fun part as with the people that you meet and the socializing that you do. We met a few people that night that I promised that I would pick them up at the beach in my speedboat the following day. Meeting a woman on the beach is wise because you get to see them in a bikini which means that they can't hide the flaws if they have any. Women are expert dressers with choosing cloths that show off their good parts of their body but hide the no so good parts of their body. Driving home a little tipsy is a good way to have a DUI because there are checkpoints everywhere but they never stop the motorcycles. Motorcycles have many advantages.

Meals

Breakfast
Egg whites
High fiber cereal
Coffee

Post-workout snack
Shake with fresh figs and apple, whey protein isolate, almond butter, ice and water

Lunch
Grilled prawns
Grilled squid
Raw oysters
White wine

Dinner
Steamed salmon
Whole grain pasta with fresh tomatoes

Nightlife
Multiple glasses of "Albarino" wine.

Exercise

Cardio
Morning wrestling, sparing and jump rope 45 min
Afternoon bike ride 15 miles
Resistance workout (body weight)
15 Sets pull-ups super-setted with pushups 15 reps

FIESTAS DEL MIRISCOS, EL GROVE

The next few days were more relaxed but we did go out on the boat quite often having fun as always. The workouts and diets were kept up which is all just part of the lifestyle I live. The days there are long and I usually use the evenings to visit my family, most notably my grandmother who is ninety-six years old and a wealth of knowledge. My Uncles and Aunts are so much fun to visit as well. In September the entire family gets together to harvest the grapes in order to make wine. I am tremendously into culture so a day out in the fields to harvest the grapes is a wonderful experience. Spain's culture is all about family and with quite a bit of socializing.

Within the next few days I was planning on going to the "Fiesta de Mariscos" in the fisherman village of "El Grove" and another day go to Portugal which is less than an hour away, especially on my "ZX" motorcycle. The "Fiesta" in "EL Grove" is a seafood festival which has many local fisherman display to sell the fresh seafood that they just caught. That evening I drove though the winding Oceanside road that leads right to "El Grove". Riding the "ZX" out there is a rush because the roads are curvy and the police are scarce. Every now and then I will get pulled over but the police are very friendly and after a short conversation I am usually on my way. Years ago whenever the police went to pull me over I would elude them with high speeds. This tactic lead nowhere because shortly after they would appear at my grandmothers house right down the road from me to ask about my whereabouts. Eluding police in small town areas is not recommended because everyone knows each other and word gets around rather quickly, especially about "el Americano" which is myself.

The seafood festival was a blast and eating an array of different seafood only made it even better. We ate clams, mussels, oysters, crab, squid, octopus, shrimp and lobster. White wine is always the beverage of preference with fish and seafood. Another cultural evening in the books!

Seafood Festival Meal

Shrimp, lobster, clams, mussels, oysters, squid and octopus steamed
White wine

Training

2 days off

VALENCA, PORTUGAL

Taking a few days off from the gym felt refreshing but waking up early in the morning I was eager to sweat so after a cup of coffee I went for a long jog along the beach. Running on sand is not only more difficult but it is much healthier and less damaging on your knees and joints. Working up a nice sweat I was feeling the "runner's high" that had been missing for a few days. The breakfast shake provided the energy that was needed for the ride to Portugal to visit my friend Luis. Wearing shorts, flip flops and a tank top I was ready for the ride with speeds in excess of 160 miles per hour! Under my helmet I always wear my headphones in order to listen to music while riding. Speeding through the port city of "Vigo" I could see the gorgeous panoramic view of the "Ria de Vigo" which is a large bay that leads into the Atlantic. Once I crossed into Portugal it was already evident that I was no longer in

Spain. The houses were less cheerful and the people seemed a bit more reserved and serious, quite the opposite of Spain.

Portugal is a bit behind the times but that is kind of a good thing because it is more traditional this way. The first town into Portugal is called "Valenca" and there is a tremendous fort that was built to protect itself from Spain. Walking through the fort was quite an experience with its cobblestone walkways that were loaded with little shops to but clothing, food and souvenirs. I stopped at a small café to eat and ordered broiled "frango" which is chicken and I also ordered a side of sautéed broccoli rabe. A glass of the local red wine went well with lunch. The wine was served to me in a "taza" which is a clay cup that almost looks like a small bowl. This was definitely and old school type of café because there was a cow and a few roaming chickens outside.

The wine was served from a huge wooden barrel with a spout sticking out of it. In other words the wine was freshly fermented in that same barrel. Lunch soon ended so I took a ride to the riverside town of "Vila Nova de Cerveira" where I went to visit my friend Luis. This little town was adorable with its cozy feel to it. Cobblestone streets all over and while having a glass of "vino Porto" which is sweet Portuguese wine we heard the beautiful church bells in the background. Right smack in the center of town was the spectacular Roman Catholic Church. Another interesting sight was the small six car ferry that crossed into Spain. The ferry was powered by a small motor that pulled onto the cable that went across the river from Portugal to Spain! This was the second smallest ferry I have ever seen, the smallest being the four car pulley driven ferry that I had traveled on when I was in Albania.

The "Port" wine was delicious and now I was off the beach town of "Caminha". The ride down was thrilling because of the twisting and banked curves right down to the very few radar traps. Nothing beats speeding on these European highways. "Caminha" was an adorable town on the Atlantic coastline. This town even had a train stop right on the beach sand! Could you believe that! That must be one unique train ride right on the sand of the coastline. The beach was pristine and the water was crystal clear and of course there were no lifeguards. Europe has more of that free and open feeling. I met two nice people on the beach. The conversation began when they noticed my foreign accent when I spoke Portuguese. The conversation led to the usual questions being where am I from and how did I get a lean and toned body. Funny isn't it but Europeans are always innocently curious about things. The three of us walked over to the local family owned restaurant for the afternoon meal. What a cool experience it was because the tables were huge so around ten of us sat next to each other on each side. Complete strangers to each other too. The food was then brought to the table in large plates along with water and wine. Everything was served "family style". Basically you had no choices of food and beverage because you ate and drank what ever the waiter brought to the table. Another cool factor was as soon as you were ready to leave you then asked for the check and the waiter would ask you what you ate and then told you the amount. In other words they didn't remember which food they served, didn't write it down and then asked you what you had. Talk about trust! Money can not buy those experiences.

Spending the rest of the afternoon walking on the beach was breathtaking. Right on the beach there was a children's park that had monkey bars and a few other slides that I could somehow use to do my workout. Doing my usual park/swim workout was done in thirty minutes which consisted of chin-ups, dips, lunges and a fast fifty meter swim in the rather large waves of the Atlantic. After exercising I enjoyed the rush by walking it off on the beach. It was time to head back home but first I stopped at a deli to have a plum and some local reduced fat goat cheese.

Once again the ride home was a blast! Listen to music while driving upwards of 160 miles per hour gives me the perfect combination of fun, fear and risk! Riding a wheelie through the toll both is a great way not to have to pay. There are cameras but they can not see your license plate when you are riding a wheelie because the plate is faced down. Saving a few bucks really isn't the reason. The rush is the main reason.

Arriving at home there were a few of the guys waiting to work out. We all hit the bags and jump roped for a few rounds. The highlight was the blackberry protein shake after the workout and a few laughs with the guys. That's what it's all about, enjoying the moment and that we most definitely we did! Another great day "in the books". No going out to clubs that night because I was exhausted plus the day was good enough so why not leave off on top!

PORTUGAL DAILY ITINERARY

Meals

Breakfast
Egg whites
Low-fat goat cheese
Coffee

Lunch
Broiled chicken with oregano
Sautéed broccoli rabe
Red wine

Afternoon meal
Whiting fish in green sauce
Tomato and onion salad
Port wine

Post workout meal
Plum
Low-fat cheese

Bedtime meal
Shake with protein, ice, water, blackberries and bran (blended)

Exercise

Cardio
Morning beach run 2 miles
Evening cardio: 3 rounds each: speed bag, jump rope, spar
Resistance exercise routine
Afternoon park workout: 10 sets dips, chin-ups, lunges, 50 yard
swim

RIA DE ALDAN, SKEET SHOOTING

This trip so far was going well. When traveling with me you are either going to love me or hate me because I'm a non-stop type of person. All day and everyday I look for the next stimulation and the next adventure. Vacationers like to relax while adventurers like risk and stimulation, of course I'm an adventurer. Whenever I travel on short trips with someone we always have a blast.

My good friend Eric is great to travel on the short trips with because we have a lot in common. We both workout, eat healthy, stay in shape, like to dress well, try new foods, new adventures on trips and we both drink but not a lot. Eric is such a good sport because regardless of the plans I make he's always up for it. However on long trips it's different. This trip began with Eric and I traveling to Pamplona, Spain to the "running of the bulls" then through the Adriatic where we then parted ways. After two weeks Eric left Croatia to return back to Miami and I returned back to Spain for another two and a half months because I have a house there in "Playa de Areas" which lies in "Galicia" which is directly on the Atlantic coast close to Portugal.

On a long trip such as this one I fall into a nice routine because I'm in the comfort of my own house that even has a gym. Being at home and at your gym is priceless because you don't even have to miss a beat. Home cooked meals and steady exercise equals staying in shape which adds to having a great vacation. Being in shape gives me the "firepower" needed to really get the most out of any trip. More nightlife, waterskiing, sightseeing and going to the beach are a result of having that "firepower" which people would love to have. Not to get off the details of this trip I woke up early again and had some breakfast at the local café. A good "carajillo" along with some fresh cured cheese and six boiled egg whites.

As soon as I ate my breakfast the day needed to be planned and this day would be different. Skeet shooting on a boat wouldn't appeal to everyone but mess and the guys like it. Pablo, Marcos, and I would go. I needed to bring three smaller gauged shotguns; a .410 gauge, a twenty-eight gauge and a twenty gauge shotgun. I also have a few twelve gauge shotguns but they are too powerful to be shooting all afternoon because the noise may scare people   and have them call the marine patrol and the more powerful weapons also hurt your shoulder more from the excessive recoil. These weapons were great gifts from kind friends of mine.   Whenever a good friend comes to visit me to spend a few weeks at the house they always insist on buying me a gift so usually an inexpensive weapon or fireworks are among my first choices.

With these weapons we would go to the "Ria de Aldan" because it was a fairly tranquil area with not too tourists. During the shooting three of us would shoot while one of us would take turns launching the disks, cans and bottles while also looking out for the marine police. The few times the marine police appeared I quickly sped away and at seventy miles per hour they wouldn't be able to catch up to my boat. From my house we bicycled to "Raxo", a small fishermen's village where I park the boat. From there our destination would be thirty minutes away. The ride there was a blast thanks to the waves we were jumping over. Once there we "set up shop" by picking a good spot and loading the weapons. Firing away the blasts could be heard miles away along the water. We had a great time and what a success it was because there were no accidents, no passing boats or seagulls were hit and there were no police in sight during the entire time.

After the nice adrenaline rush it was time to eat so we pulled up close to the shore, dropped the anchor and walked waist deep to shore where there was a beach front tavern that was serving food. We could smell the sardines being grilled. I ordered food for everyone by walking into the kitchen and asking the cook to prepare our food without salt or grease. He cooked a delicious combination of sardines and veal along with a tasty salad and wine. The meal ended and no explanation was needed why I ordered without salt because the cook noticed the muscle in my arm and realized that is how I had it, from eating right. Nevertheless I blushed a little because I am rather shy whenever I receive a compliment.

As soon we got home it was time for a game of handball because in my backyard there's a handball court. After the warm up game of two on two we began a new workout, the "four minute set workout" which I had learned from my good friends in the U.S. Ray and Nabil. It's a great workout with a lot of good sweating followed by a refreshing protein shake made with nuts and fruit. Exercising shortly prior to going out is a fantastic way to "hit the scene" because you're already "warmed up" to begin socializing enabling your works to flow and your personality to be at its best. Driving my motorcycle, the Kawasaki "ZX" is the best way to go out to the pier which is packed with partygoers because the traffic is dense and parking is difficult which none of this applies to being on a motorcycle because you squeeze between the traffic and park right in front of the nightclubs. The other benefit is motorcycled usually aren't stopped at DUI checkpoints.

Arriving to the scene was intense because all you see is ancient architecture, cobblestone streets, vibrant street life and well dressed attractive people, a winning combination. Running into a few friends and starting off with a few drinks started the evening before going to the "Dux" which is "the" place to go with its lavish décor. There is always a line to get into "Dux" but I'm able to circumvent it by entering through the "VIP" entrance. "VIP" status was given to me because many of the nightclub's security guards either work out at my gym, have broken up a fight of mine during my earlier years or know me from either waterskiing on my boat or motocross, quad or motorcycle riding. Via either scenario the security guards treat me like family nevertheless.

The "Dux" was at its best that evening. After a few drinks and socializing with an attractive olives skinned brunette by the name of "Montse" I already knew I was in for a great evening. "Montse" was an educated Mediterranean looking young woman. She really appreciated the time with me because she was laughing at either my jokes or at me which is quite alright because when a women laugh a lot with you is a tell tale sign that likes you. Women really like a guy who can make them laugh. However do not buy joke books and carry them around with you because your humor must be natural and never scripted.

The evening went extremely well with "Montse" and riding a few "wheelies" on the motorcycle while driving her home was the icing on the cake. She really appreciated my uniqueness. By no means am I a Casanova because many of women have told me to "get lost" while trying to talk to them. But with Montse it all went well.

RIA DE ALDAN

Meals

Breakfast
Freshly cured lamb cheese
6 Boiled hard boiled egg whites
"Carajillo" (espresso coffee mixed with brandy)

Lunch
Grilled sardines and veal
Green salad with extra virgin olive oil and balsamic vinegar

"Albarino" white wine

Post workout meal
Shake: whey protein isolate, cashews, figs, oat bran, water, ice, water

Nightlife
2 Shots of "Patron" tequila with lemon and salt

Exercise

Shoulders
1 straight 4 minute set of each exercise (these sets are to be performed with a stopwatch for 4 straight minutes with breaks up to no more than 20 seconds)
Dumbbell lateral raises
Bent over cable lateral raises
Dumbbell front press
Smith machine front press

Abs
Reverse crunches

Cardio
Playing a few games of handball
Home Made Wine

Now that the summer crowd was gone my next adventure would be to help my extended family pick the grapes from the vine in order to make the wine. My uncles and cousins have plenty of land that they use to grow grapes and making home brewed wine is like a national pastime in Spain. Wine is everywhere there so farmers tend to boast about how good their wine is. My family is always glad to have me help out especially with the heavy work of loading and unloading the buckets of grapes into the cars and trucks. My family is under the impression that my body was developed from hard labor and not weights. It's kind of funny but I'm always pleased to be of assistance to them. It's the least that I could do for anyone that was always so good to me while growing up. Before heading out to the vineyards my day began with a healthy breakfast consisting of home made salt-free whole grain bread, home made blackberry preserves, café con leche and a "tortilla Espanola" which is a Spanish omelet made with eggs and potatoes but instead I made it with egg whites and sweet potatoes. An hour later my friends called me to play indoor soccer. The indoor soccer field was in the small mountain town called "Bordones" which lies a few miles up from the beach.

Riding there on bicycle was a convenient way for me to warm up for the game. As soon as I got there the game was to be relocated onto the beach because the gym was closed. The beach was gorgeous but playing soccer on the beach is a lot more tiring but that's ok because a harder workout is always better. The game was so much fun and at the half time we jumped into the ocean to cool off. When the second half and the game ended I wanted to drink water so I walked over to a group of huge rocks right on the beach that had a natural fresh water stream shooting up about two feet high.

Coming home I was exhausted so a shake with melon was the next meal. Forty-five minutes later it was time to meet the family at the vineyards. Helping my "Tio Claudio", "Tia Ysolina", "Tio Manolo" and cousin "Elsa" was a lot of fun because in Spain the family shows there love for one another by working together. And after working together everyone eats together. I find this very endearing. There is nothing like that "old world" European culture. It really is priceless. The food we ate wasn't the healthiest but every now and them you need to splurge a little plus eating over a Spaniard's house will be very difficult not to gorge yourself with delicious food. We ate "empanada de pulpo", "empanada de calamares" and "Empanada de atun". These were pizza like thin baked bread with either tuna, squid or octopus.

That evening the guys came over to train and it was leg day which tends to be the least desirable of all the muscles to train because it is usually the most difficult. It was rough but we finished within forty-five minutes as usual. Finishing off with a shake made with macadamia nuts and grapes was the post-workout meal. Soon after I went into the Jacuzzi for a while because I was exhausted from such a full day of work, excitement, exercise and fulfillment. This evening my body was too tired for the nightlife and club "scene". Spain's nightlife is among the best in the world so that even if I miss a night or two of partying that's ok because it is so easy to make up for. Whether it being a Monday or Saturday evening there is always somewhere to go that has a crowd of people.

DAILY ITINERARY

Meals

Breakfast
Café con leche
Unsalted whole grain bread with strawberry preserves
Egg white and sweet potato omelet

Snack
Protein shake: whey protein isolate melon, oats, ice and water

Lunch
Tuna empanada
Squid empanada
Octopus empanada

Post-workout snack
Shake: whey protein isolate, macadamia nuts, melon, ice and water

Exercise

Legs
Sets are 4 minutes non-stop
Leg extensions
Leg curls
Lunges
Front squats
Individual leg hamstring curl

Cardio
Beach soccer 45 minutes

LA CORUNA

Now that the vacation was winding down I needed one last weekend away in the city of "La Coruna" where my mother's family is from. First I needed to pull my boat out from the water into the garage for winter storing along with the quad and motorcycles. That's a full day of work and having several toys can sometimes be a headache because of all the time that's needed for the upkeep of the vehicles. Tidying up in "Playa de Areas" took several hours because winterizing everything is time consuming and I wouldn't be back for at least a year. Saying goodbye to everyone isn't easy especially for me because I'm a bit sensitive and I tend to shed a few tears after saying goodbye to loved ones.

Driving to "La Coruna" was so much fun because the roads really are beautiful and well engineered so driving my rental car, a turbo diesel Ford Focus at full speed which was 115 miles per hour made the journey even more fun. Down hill I reached 125 mph. Back home in the U.S. I have a modified BMW M6 which at nearly 600 horsepower and six-speed manual transmission would be a total thrill to drive along Spain's highways. I have reached 175 mph with it in the U.S. but that's very risky for me considering that I haven't received any points in the last ten years which brings me down to fifty-three points! And that's not including the points I've had with my out of state drivers licenses.

As soon as I arrived to the city first I visited the family and went out with them for some "tapas" right on the "calle Real" which is the main street in La Coruna. We ate a variety of "tapas", they were "pulpo", "calamares", "callos", "navajas", "gambas" and "langostinos" which were a combination of octopus, squid, tripe, razor clams, shrimp and prawns. All of the food was healthy minus the tripe but it all tasted great and enjoying myself with the family was the best part. No training that day and the next morning I was flying back to the U.S. Another summer gone by with some great memories in it. This three month vacation was spectacular because I had a great time and I stayed in shape.

My three month vacation was a journey and it all started July 9th, the day after I had an MMA fight in New York City. The next day Eric and I were on route to the "running of the bulls" in Pamplona Spain, then to Venice Italy, Corfu Greece, Saranda Beach and Tirana Albania, Budva Beach and Kotor Montenegro, Bosnia then Dubrovnik and Split Croatia where Eric headed back to the U.S. and from Zagreb Croatia I continued my journey to Barcelona , Madrid, my beach house in "Playa de Areas" where I stayed for two and a half months, then to visit my Mother's family in "La Coruna" then on a day trip to northern Portugal and finally it was back to the land of opportunity, the U.S.

Meals "Tapas"

"Gambas al ajillo" Shrimp with garlic
 "Langostinos a la plancha" Grilled prawns
"Trips" Tripe with chickpeas and sausage
"Pulpo a la Gallega" Octopus with olive oil and paprika
"Calamares a la Romana" Squid with tomato sauce

Plan Your Next Trip or Dream

All in all I am totally grateful to have had these priceless traveling experiences. Often I reminisce about the great life I have been living so I've decided to share it with you.

This book is my second of several more to come teaches you that all of our dreams are possible so any thoughts and ideas you may have to just go for it and never look back! Life is short and youth is even shorter so whatever you're thinking of doing, do it now! Time waits for no one! In 1990 I ate a fortune cookie that had the note inside "life to you is one big dashing adventure" then fifteen years later after eating another fortune cookie it had the same fortune and true it was! Never did I forget that fortune from 1990 and I kept thinking that that's how my life was; a dashing adventure! So make your life too a dashing adventure.

Go out and go after it, be spontaneous, follow your dreams, your goals and don't wait for tomorrow because it may never come. Don't be a "could've, would've, should've type of person. Don't be a "why" person and instead be a "why not" person and go for it and now! Not tomorrow! Life's all about timing and chances so believe in yourself because when you "believe you shall achieve"!

REGIONAL FOODS

Spain

To talk of a single Spanish cuisine wouldn't be very accurate in our country. You would have to talk about an ensemble of diverse and independent regional cuisines. These cuisines are a
reflection of the history and culture of the people and villages of Spain.

Ours is a varied cuisine with some common points connecting it. Just to give some examples, we'll say that roasted meat is plentiful on the plateau, rice is typical of Spanish Levante and foods fried in olive oil are typically Andalusian; but, this would simplify things too much. Besides local dishes, dishes from other parts of the country are prepared in most Spanish homes.

Despite the aforementioned variety, there are some common features that characterize our entire territory:

The use of olive oil as the basic culinary fat - both uncooked as well as for fried foods and sauce bases.

The use of onion and garlic as basic condiments.

Sofrito (fried onion, garlic and tomato) as a base for many dishes.

Bread with meals.

Soups as the first course.

Plenty of salads, especially in the summer.

Having wine or beer with meals.

Fruit as dessert or a dairy product (normally yogurt). Sweets (cakes or pastries) are often reserved for special days.

Among the large number of dishes that make up the broad and diverse Spanish recipe collection, there are a few that could be considered common to the entire territory. Some of them have a known origin and continue to be associated to certain regions even though they are prepared throughout the country such as the Spanish omelet or tortilla de patatas, paella, ratatouille, gazpacho, fried breadcrumbs and cured meats (Serrano ham, chorizo, blood sausage) as well as the different cheeses (there is no region without their own). Dishes with legumes as the base (lentils, chickpeas, beans, etc.) are frequent as are stews; however, each region places their own spin on these dishes. We mustn't forget the bread and the many ways to make it leading to very different varieties in each region. And, above all, the various regions most coincide on desserts and sweets: cream caramel, custard, rice pudding, torrijas (bread soaked in milk and fried), fairy cake and churros are some of the most common.

Likewise, you can't just talk about Spanish wine. Using the plural form is just as necessary as when discussing the gastronomy.

Wine is part of a thousand-year-old tradition in Spain ever since the introduction of the vine and its conversion into wine by the Phoenicians.

The variety of wines that can be found throughout the Spanish territory is immense. Each Autonomous Region features several winemaking areas of interest (called Denominations of Origin) where excellent quality, famous wine is produced such as Rioja, Ribera del Duero, Jerez, Peneds... But, other regions that are less well-known abroad also make great quality wines with an interesting present and fantastic future. There are even wines that do not pertain to any D.O. that can be of great quality and for this reason, they have been granted a geographic indication known as Regional Wines or Vinos de la Tierra.

Even people who do not usually drink wine, sometimes drink it in a form known as "tinto de verano", combined with lemonade; or in sangria, one of the most typical Spanish beverages known worldwide.

Portugal

In the 15th century, Prince Henry the Navigator ordered his explorers to bring back to Portugal any exotic fruits, nuts, and plants from new lands. As a result, the Age of Discovery dramatically affected cooking in Portugal and around the world.

Tomatoes and potatoes were taken to Europe, Brazilian pineapples were introduced to the Azores, Brazilian chili peppers grew in Angola, African coffee was transplanted to Brazil (today producing about half of the world's supply), Brazilian cashews landed in Africa and India, and tea was introduced to Europeans. Today, the Portuguese fondness for certain ingredients like cinnamon or curry powder for example, is also a legacy from this time. But other cultures had been introducing new foods to Portugal for centuries before that. The Romans (who aimed to make the Iberian Peninsula the granary of Rome) brought wheat and introduced onions, garlic, olives, and grapes. Later, the Moors were the first to plant rice, introduced figs, planted groves of lemons and oranges, and covered the Algarve province with almond trees.

Today, naturally, Portuguese food varies from region to region, but fresh fish and shellfish are found on virtually every menu. The national dish is "bacalhau," dried, salted cod. The Portuguese have been obsessed with it since the early 16th century, when their fishing boats reached Newfoundland. The sailors salted and sun-dried their catch to make it last the long journey home, and today there are said to be 365 different ways of preparing it, one
for each day of the year.

Grilled sardines and horse mackerel are also popular in the coastal towns, and a mixture of other types of fish is put into a stew called "Caldeirada."

The country is full of specialty seafood restaurants, many with artistic displays of lobsters, shrimp, oysters, and crabs. To try a mixture of these, have the rich seafood rice, "arroz de marisco."

Another national dish, but made with meat, is "cozido à portuguesa," a thick stew of vegetables with various kinds of meat. The favorite kind is pork, cooked and served in a variety of ways. Roast suckling pig ("leitão assado") is popular in the north of the country, as are pork sausages called "chouriço" or "linguiça."

Typical of Porto is tripe with haricot beans. It is not to everyone's taste, but has been Porto's most famous dish since Henry the Navigator sent a vessel to conquer Ceuta in Morocco and the people of Porto slaughtered all their livestock to provision the crew, keeping just the intestines for themselves. They have been known as "tripeiros" or "tripe eaters" ever since.

Breakfast is traditionally just coffee and a bread roll, but lunch is a big affair, often lasting up to two hours. It is served between noon and 2 o'clock or between 1 and 3 o'clock, and dinner is generally served late, after 8 o'clock. There are usually three courses, often including soup. The most common soup is "caldo verde," with potato, shredded cabbage, and chunks of sausage.

The most typical desserts are cinnamon-flavored rice pudding, flan, and caramel custard, but they also often include a variety of cheese. The most common varieties are made from sheep or goat's milk, and the most popular is "queijo da serra" from the region of Serra da Estrela.

Many of the country's outstanding pastries were created by nuns in the 18th century, which they sold them as a means of supplementing their incomes. Many of their creations have
interesting names like "barriga de freira" (nun's belly), "papos de anjo" (angel's chests), and "toucinho do céu" (bacon from heaven). A particularly delicious pastry is "pastel de nata," a small custard tart sprinkled with cinnamon.

Before any meal at a restaurant in Lisbon or elsewhere in Portugal, try the bread placed on the table—Portuguese bread is delicious.

Italy

Italian cuisine is one of the most popular in the world. There are so many Italian recipes that you will find several variations of the same dish. For example lasagna made in the north of Italy is very different from the one made in the south. Famous Italian recipes are for pasta, pizza, seafood, poultry, meat and vegetable dishes. Desserts are also very famous. You will find more seafood dishes coming from the coastal areas of Italy such as Naples, Venice, Genova, etc. Piedmont is famous for his meats (often eaten raw) and truffles. Tuscany is also famous for meat and game as well as cacciucco (seafood stew) from Livorno.

An Italian meal

A formal meal in Italy is a succession of courses, with no main course, starting with an antipasto, followed by a first course (primo) of either pasta, risotto, or soup; and a second course (secondo) of meat, poultry, or fish, accompanied by one or two vegetable side dishes (contorni). Then there is a salad (insalata), sometimes cheese, and the meal ends with fruit or dessert (dolce) or both.

Antipasto never played an important part in Italian eating. Not long ago it consisted of only a few slices of prosciutto or salame, and these are still the favorites. Antipasto is meant only to whet the appetite, so do not make too much. For most people in Italy the first course is the most important, and pasta is the favorite food. Although most people prefer the simplest treatment - olive oil and garlic with fresh raw tomato and basil or a dressing of butter melted with sage leaves, sprinkled with freshly grated black pepper and parmigiano reggiano - the versatility of pasta is extraordinary. Risotto, gnocchi and other rice dishes are also versatile. Soups can be a meal in themselves or light and delicate.

With so much coast Italy has a wide range of fish and seafood. Until recently fish was considered to be a Friday dish only, and not grand enough to serve to guests, but now it is one of the most popular foods. Meat and poultry dishes are mostly grills, roasts, and stews; there are lovely game dishes, and offal is particularly good. Egg dishes and vegetable dishes can also be served as a second course. Vegetable dishes are an important part of every meal, so make good use of the repertoire. Salad can be a green salad or cooked vegetables dressed with olive oil and lemon juice.

Cheese is served at the end of the meal in northern Italy, especially in Piedmont, but not usually in the south. At home, dessert is generally fruit, sweets being reserved for special and festive occasions. After fruit or dessert, strong black coffee from a high or after dinner roast may be served in small cups, and perhaps followed with brandy or grappa, an amaro (bitter), anise-flavored sambuca or a sweet wine such as vin santo, accompanied by pastries or biscotti with almonds for dunking.

Greece

Want to know what Greek people eat? If you are visiting Greece on holiday or vacation you are in for a culinary treat.

Situated in south-eastern Europe, Greece is a sun kissed land with an all year round temperate climate which provides an abundance of fresh vegetables, fruits and herbs to compliment their excellent cuisine.

Nowhere in Greece is much further from the sea than around 80 miles, so fish as well as meat plays a central role in Greek cuisine.

Sheep and Goats thrive on the precipitous slopes of the mountains in Greece and their milk makes the wonderful Feta cheese, so much part of the cuisine.

Of the many salads containing fresh vegetables and herbs, the Greek salad is most famed in the cuisine of Greece, with its layers of juicy onions, sun ripened tomatoes and green leaves, with generous pieces of Feta cheese which is dressed in the wonderful oil taken from the olives which grow in abundance across the hills and plains of Greece.

Lamb plays a principal role in the cuisine of Greece and is often spit roasted during festivals, of which there are many as Greeks love to celebrate together.

The lamb is also slow cooked in the oven, stewed, or casseroled. Lamb Kleftika, a popular dish in the cuisine of Greece, is slow cooked in a packet of paper with scented herbs and often topped with Feta.

Moussaka is perhaps one of the most famous dishes in the cuisine of Greece with its layers of garlic scented minced meat sauce and egg plant topped with a succulent savory custard.

With hundreds of islands and so much coastline, the cuisine in Greece contains many wonderful fish and shellfish dishes cooked in a variety of methods from simply grilled and served on a bed of salad leaves and drizzled with oil or cooked in a stew.

Kalamaria (squid) is a favored fish dish in the cuisine of Greece and Taramosalata is a popular fish roe spread.

Another popular dish in the cuisine of Greece is Dolmades which is vine leaves stuffed with rice and meat and soaked in oil.

The cheeses of Greece play a prominent role in its cuisine and cheese pies are an every day favorite with the cheese cooked in crumble fila pastry packets. Apart from Feta, Kasseri is a creamy cheese which is popular and Kefalotiri which is hard and salty and hence ideal for grating.

The people of Greece are fond of their sweet cuisine dishes and Baklava is one of the most famous with its layers of fila pastry, nuts and sticky honey sauce.

As far as drinks which accompany the cuisine in Greece are concerned, Ouzo is a famous liqueur which is clear and flavored with aniseed. Retsina is a red or white wine flavored with pine Resin.

Albania

The cuisine of Albania, as with most Mediterranean and Balkan nations, has been strongly influenced by its long history. The territory of Albania has been occupied by Greece, Italy and the Ottoman Turks and each group has left its mark on Albanian cuisine.

Milk from goats and ewes is made into kos and many varieties of cheeses. Oranges, lemons, and figs are the main available fruits; some grapes and wild berries are made into fermented beverages. Mixed garden vegetables are used seasonally and as available. These include: cucumbers, onions, peppers, eggplants, zucchini, marrows, okra, squash (kungull), potatoes, and tomatoes. With the establishment of canneries, there has been a gradual increase in the consumption of canned fruits and vegetables in the Albanian food. The favored meats are lamb and mutton and sometimes chicken. Liver is considered a delicacy Albanian food. Meats are usually prepared in types of stews or as pilafs with rice, or skewered and roasted over open fires. There is also a variety of nuts grown locally: walnuts, almonds, pine nuts, and hazelnuts. These may be used as nibbles, crushed (sometimes with garlic), and as sauces over meats and/or vegetables. The most successful crops of the Albanian farmer have for centuries been grains. Predominantly corn, but also wheat, rye, oats, and barley are harvested. These grains have been used to produce a variety of flours for breads that are consumed mainly in coastal areas and cities. But the main type of bread - indeed the main food - is a flat pancake-shaped corn bread broken into pieces and enjoyed with kos or cheese. Olive oil is the main type of fat used everywhere. Albanians enjoy very sweet and rich desserts made with nuts and syrupy sauces. The combination of thin, crisp pastries (identical to the Greek phyllo) with nuts, sugar or honey, cinnamon, and cloves, and finished with a heavy syrup, or very sweet puddings, are as beloved by the Albanians as they are by the Turks and Greeks. People who favor very sweet desserts will almost certainly also enjoy highly seasoned Albanian food, and the Albanians are no exception. Generous portions of garlic and onions, tart touches of lemon juice or lemon grating, and the more subtle enhancement of dill and parsley as well as cinnamon and cloves waft through Albanian food. The combination of crushed or chopped nuts with garlic and oil, to be served with greens or chicken, as well as the combination of nuts and raisins either for nibbling or as part of exotic sauces, are all typically Albanian food.

The main meal is lunch which is usually accompanied by a salad of fresh vegetables, such as tomatoes, cucumbers, green peppers, and olives dressed with olive oil, vinegar and salt. Seafood specialties are common in the coastal areas of Durres, Vlore and Sarande.

Some of their specialties are: Fërgesë of Tirana with veal a dish made with veal, cottage or feta cheese, onions and spices, Qofte Te Ferguara fried meatballs made of lamb, beef or chicken, Tave Kosi baked lamb with yogurt sauce, Gjelle Me Arra veal or chicken with walnuts, Byrek Shqiptar Me Perime an Albanian vegetable pie with phylo dough, spinach, feta cheese and chopped green onions, Tave Me Prech leek casserole baked with ground beef, Jamime Fasule or bean yahni soup with white beans, onion, tomato sauce, chopped parsley, mint and spices, Turli Perimesh a main dish of mixed vegetables such as peppers, eggplant, okra, zucchini, potatoes etc. with chopped onions, tomatoes and parsley added, Mish Qingjji Me Barbunja veal with large lima beans, Eomlek rabbit casserole with onions and wine, Qafte Me Veze Dhe Limon ground lamb meatballs in an egg and lemon sauce, Speca Te Mbushura stuffed peppers with or without ground meat, rice, chopped dill, parsley and tomato puree and as an appetizer Tarator fried eggplant, zucchini and green peppers with plain yogurt.

Montenegro

Traditional Montenegrin Meals

Kacamak – is a mushy, strong meal which made of wheat, buckwheat, barley, or corn flour and which is being served with cheese and sour milk. Wet "kacamak" is called the one to which the cheese is added, or "kajmak" and which is being stirred for a long time with a special wooden spoon. The taste is even better, and people in the villages prefer it because it gives them the energy which they are using in hard labor. It is found in the offer of every national restaurant. Kacamak made of potato is maybe to most interesting variant of this meal.

Cicvara – with this meal usually white cooked potato and sour milk are being served. Young cow's cheese or "kajmak" are mixed with flour while the grease is released. It is a meal of high
energetic value, of pleasant taste – it literarily melts in your mouth.

Popara – with mixing of bread with milk, oil and cheese you get an interesting and cheap meal which is deeply seated in the Montenegrin cuisine.

Cooked potato – is an easy and favorite meal which is accompanied with the cheese, and sour cabbage. It is simply prepared – with a half an hour of cooking of potato.

Thick soups – thick soups in Montenegro are usually prepared with noodles, potato or vegetables. Especially interesting thick soap is the one made of nettle, and almost every thick soup included the cooked fresh meat, so they are extremely nourishing and rich.

"Rastan" – a strong meal made of local vegetable from the family of cabbages, it is cooked with white potato and with a lot of spices.

"Japraci" – is an extremely rich and nourishing meal. In a kilo of "rastan" and half a kilo of young cow's meet rice, pepper, and even dry meat are added. With cooking the grease is being released, and the meal gets the right flavor. Sarma, stuffed peppers, stew, pilaf etc are still just some meals which beside in Montenegro are characteristic for some other countries on the Balkans. Each of these meals carries a small but significant part of Montenegro in themselves, so we are warmly recommending them during your staying in these areas.

Montenegrin lamb in milk – is a real specialty. From about 2 kg of meat which are being cooked in domestic milk with the addition of spices and potato, you can serve 8 persons, so especially in the north, this meals is being prepared during some solemn occasions.

Sausage – is prepared by drying, most often in Njegusi, with a special technique. It is extremely tasty and strong.

Prsuta (smoked ham) – most famous "prsut", the one from Njegusi, excels with quality eve compared to the Italian producers. It is the meat of which people take care day and night, while it is dried exclusively on beech logs, for several months. It is served with the domestic, most often grape brandy, and with the dry cheese from Njegusi.

Lamb made under iron pan – When we are talking about the meals made under the iron pan it would be interesting to mention the very process of preparing. The meals made under the iron pan are by far more tasteful than all other meals because they are put under an iron pan the so-called "sac", which is then covered by ember and ashes. In this way, the aroma is being kept, and the meal is equally fried in a natural way. Lamb, for e.g. is most tasteful if it is prepared in this way. Montenegrin national restaurants prepare it in this way even today.

Popeci from Podgorica – it is interestingly arranged meal: in a steak made from veal's meat you roll in a piece of cheese or old "kajmak" and a piece of "prsut". Then you further fry that roll in deep oil, and you get a meal of great juicy and rich interiors and of tasteful and crunchy exterior.

The food from the grill – Montenegrins are known as great lovers of the grill; especially the tasty "cevapi" (kebab) and grilled meat patty which go excellently with onion. Those are two most popular meals with younger population and they are found in the offer of fast food restaurants.

Bosnia

Cuisine of Bosnia and Herzegovina is balanced between Western and Eastern influences. Bosnian food is closely related to Turkish, Middle Eastern and other Mediterranean cuisines. However, due to years of Austrian rule and influence, there are also many culinary influences from Central Europe.

Bosnian cuisine uses many spices, but usually in moderate quantities. Most dishes are light, as they are cooked in lots of water; the sauces are fully natural, consisting of little more than the natural juices of the vegetables in the dish. Typical ingredients include tomatoes, potatoes, onions, garlic, bell peppers, cucumbers, carrots, cabbage, mushrooms, spinach, zucchini, dried and fresh beans, plums, milk, paprika and cream called pavlaka. Typical meat dishes include primarily beef and lamb. Some local specialties are cevapcici, burek, dolma, sarma, pilav, goulash, ajvar and a whole range of Eastern sweets. The best local wines come from Herzegovina where the climate is suitable for growing grapes. Plum or apple Rakija is produced in Bosnia (region).

Bosnians have a special way of cooking; traditional meals are very appreciated especially in the old town. In the big cities like Sarajevo, Zenica, and Tuzla, you can find restaurants with specifically Mediterranean cuisine. A traditional Bosnian meal cannot exclude meat. Traditional desserts include milk and milk products like cream. Baklava is a traditional dessert which contains sweet nuts and honey in pastry. In Bosnia, hamburgers called pljeskavica are made in a special type of bread named pita bread. Bosnian salads are generally prepared with mixed tomatoes, lettuce, onion, pepper and cheese. Many pickled foods are served as salads for a meal, such as pickled cucumbers, tomatoes, peppers, onions. In the Bosnian cuisine the salads are usually accompanying the main dish but it also can be eaten separated. The most frequent type of meat consumed by Bosnians is beef. Bosnians prefer smoked meat: smoked ribs, smoked neck or smoked sausages. They serve smoked meat uncooked on a platter or they fry it on a grill and serve it with boiled vegetables like beans and potatoes. But more common meat dishes are served with mashed or fried potatoes. Other important dishes that include meat are filovane paprike, made of fried peppers stuffed with minced meat and spices, and japrak, which is cabbage rolls stuffed with beef meat and rice.

Croatia

Typical Croatian food is normally extension of peasant food, which is easy to prepare yet delicious. As anywhere else in the world in Croatia too neighboring countries has influenced its cuisine. So while people from the Croatia's Adriatic areas eat food very similar to Italian cuisine, in northern Croatia dishes are similar to those of central Europe or Austro-Hungarian.

Because of the cuisine's heterogeneity it is also known as cuisine of the regions. Its modern roots date back to Proto-Slavic and ancient periods and the differences in the selection of foodstuffs and forms of cooking are most notable between those on the mainland and those in coastal regions. Mainland cuisine is more characterized by Proto-Slavic and the more recent contacts with Hungarian, Viennese and Turkish cuisines while the coastal areas have tremendous influence of Greek, Roman and Illyrian as well as Italian and French way of cooking.

Like in all other parts of the world, every holiday in this country also has a typical dish associated with it. Hot-pepper-flavored sausages or Kulen are eaten during the harvesting seasons, goose is laid on the table on St. Martin s Day, turkey and other fowl, as well as sarma (meat-stuffed cabbage leaves), are served on Christmas Day. While pork and potato stew is eaten on pilgrimages and at fairs; cod is prepared for Christmas Eve and Good Friday; pork is eaten on New Year's Day and doughnuts are an integral part of carnival festivities. In the southern parts of the country they prepare a similar fried sweet dish known as hrostule. During Easter's, ham and boiled eggs with green vegetables are served while desserts comprise traditional cakes called Pincas.

At weddings, a variety of dishes with dozens of cakes and biscuits are served, including breskvice, shortbread bear paws, gingerbread biscuits and plain fritters are served.

The favorite meals on all occasions include spit-roasted lamb and suckling pig, grilled fish, calamari, barbecue dishes like raznjici, cevapcici and mixed grill - prosciutto and sheep's cheese, or smoked ham and cottage cheese with sour cream, fish stew, and venison.

Croatian people also use a food enhancer called Vegeta (vegetable seasoning) to flavor their dishes. This product is made in Croatia and is available in Polish and German delicatessens in
Europe and America.

With such a huge array of food and cuisine, Croatia also has a broad palette of high quality wines, brandies, fruit juices, beers and mineral water. In fact there are up to 700 wines with protected geographic origin. In the south, people drink bevanda with their food. Bevanda is heavy, richly flavored red wine mixed with plain water and in northwestern regions it is gemisht dry, flavored wines mixed with mineral water.